Preventing Childhood Obesity in Early Care and Education Programs

Selected Standards from
*Caring for Our Children: National Health and Safety Performance Standards; Guidelines for Early Care and Education Programs, 3rd Edition**

Developed by

American Academy of Pediatrics

American Public Health Association

National Resource Center for Health and Safety in Child Care and Early Education
2010

Support for this project was provided by the
Department of Health and Human Services,
Health Resources and Services Administration,
Maternal and Child Health Bureau
(Cooperative Agreement # U46MC09810)

Funding for the pre-released selected standards,
Preventing Childhood Obesity in Early Care and Education Programs, was provided by the
Department of Health and Human Services,
Administration for Children and Families,
Child Care Bureau

**Caring for Our Children, 3rd Edition* Comprehensive Set of Standards will be published in 2011

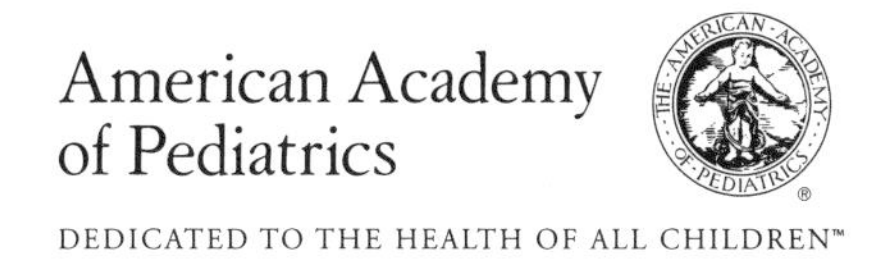

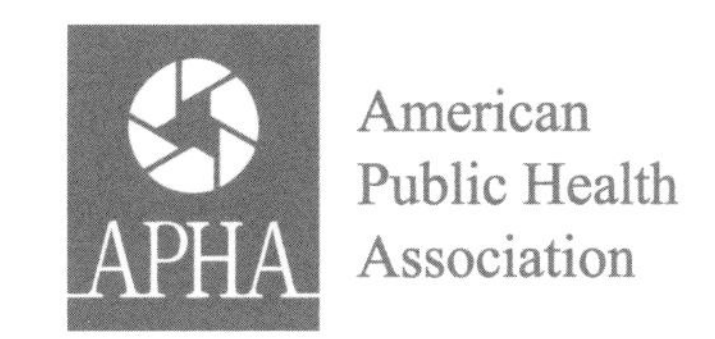

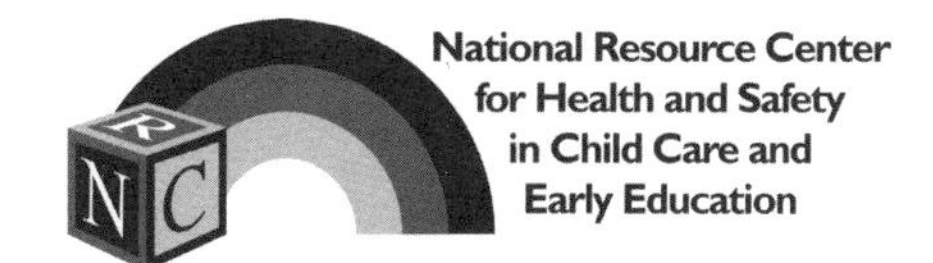

American Academy of Pediatrics ISBN: 978-1-58110-553-7
Library of Congress Control Number: 2010912446

American Public Health Association

National Resource Center for Health and Safety in Child Care and Early Education

Second Printing, September 2010.

The National Standards are for reference purposes only and shall not be used as a substitute for medical consultation, nor be used to authorize actions beyond a person's licensing, training, or ability.

Suggested Citation format:
American Academy of Pediatrics, American Public Health Association, and National Resource Center for Health and Safety in Child Care and Early Education. 2010. *Preventing Childhood Obesity in Early Care and Education: Selected Standards from Caring for Our Children: National Health and Safety Performance Standards; Guidelines for Early Care and Education Programs, 3rd Edition.* http://nrckids.org/CFOC3/PDFVersion/preventing_obesity.pdf

Editorial Consultant: Virginia R. Torrey, BS

Design and Typesetting: Susan Paige Lehtola, BBA

Research Assistant: Garrett Risley, BS

MA0579

TABLE OF CONTENTS

Please Note: Caregiver/Teacher professional development in nutrition and physical activity will be covered in the Staffing Section and facility requirements for indoor and outdoor play areas will be covered in the Playground Section of the comprehensive set of *Caring for Our Children* Standards to be released 2011.

FOREWORD

The American Academy of Pediatrics (AAP), the American Public Health Association (APHA), the National Resource Center for Health and Safety in Child Care and Early Education (NRC), and the U.S. Department of Health and Human Services, Health Resources and Services Administration, Maternal and Child Health Bureau (MCHB) are pleased to pre-release *Preventing Childhood Obesity in Early Care and Education Programs,* a set of national standards describing evidence-based best practices in nutrition, physical activity, and screen time for early care and education programs. The standards are for ALL types of early care and education settings – centers and family child care homes. These updated standards will be a part of the third edition of the new comprehensive *Caring for Our Children: National Health and Safety Performance Standards; Guidelines for Early Care and Education Programs, Third Edition* (*CFOC, 3rd Ed.*) to be released in 2011*. The standards support key national campaigns for early development of healthy lifestyle habits such as *Let's Move* (1) and *Healthy Weight Initiative* (2), and specifically assist early care and education programs with the development and implementation of best practices, procedures, and policies to instill healthy behavior and healthy lifestyle choices in our youngest children in direct support of the prevention of obesity.

The Steering Committee of *CFOC 3rd Ed.* gives special thanks to the Nutrition Technical Panel Chair Catherine Cowell, PhD, and Technical Panel members for the extraordinary effort, expertise, and time spent to accelerate this subset of standards for early release to help guide national discussions, and most importantly, to serve as guidelines for early care and education caregivers/teachers and the families of children in these settings. Gratitude also goes to the Child Development, Children with Special Health Care Needs, Environmental Quality, General Health, Infectious Diseases, Injury Prevention, Organization and Administration, and Staff Health Technical Panels that provided expertise on selected nutrition, physical activity, and screen time standards and to the forty-two stakeholders from the field who reviewed the standards for practicality, accuracy, and usefulness.

Caring For Our Children, Third Edition Steering Committee Members:

Danette Glassy, MD, FAAP (Co-Chair)
Jonathan B. Kotch, MD, MPH, FAAP (Co-Chair)
Phyllis Stubbs-Wynn, MD, MPH
Marilyn J. Krajicek, EdD, RN, FAAN
Barbara U. Hamilton, MA

Caring For Our Children, Third Edition Nutrition Technical Panel Members:

Catherine Cowell, PhD (Chair)
Donna Blum-Kemelor, MS, RD, LD
Robin Brocato, MHS
Kristen Copeland, MD, FAAP
Suzanne Haydu, MPH, RD
Janet Hill, MS, RD, IBCLC
Susan L. Johnson PhD
Ruby Natale, PhD, PsyD
Sara Benjamin Neelon, PhD, MPH, RD
Jeanette Panchula, BSW, RN, PHN, IBCLC
Shana Patterson, RD
Barbara Polhamus, PhD, MPH, RD
Susan Schlosser, MS, RD
Denise Sofka, MPH, RD
Jamie Stang, PhD, MPH, RD

AAP, APHA, and MCHB Final Manuscript Reviewers:

Noel Chavez, PhD, RD, LDN
Elaine Donoghue, MD, FAAP
Gilbert L. Fuld, MD, FAAP
Joseph F. Hagan, Jr., MD, FAAP
Sandra G. Hassink, MD, FAAP
Geraldine Henchy, MPH, RD
V. Faye Jones, MD, PhD, MSPH, FAAP
Janet Silverstein, MD, FAAP
Denise Sofka, MPH, RD
Nicolas Stettler, MD, MSCE, FAAP
Jeanne VanOrsdal, MEd

1. The White House. 2010. *Let's move campaign.* http://www.letsmove.gov/.
2. U.S. Department of Health and Human Services. 2010. *The Surgeon General's Vision for a Healthy and Fit Nation.* Rockville, MD: U.S. DHHS, OSG. http://www.surgeongeneral.gov/library/obesityvision/obesityvision2010.pdf.

**Caring for Our Children: National Health and Safety Performance Standards; Guidelines for Early Care Education Programs, Third Edition* (*CFOC 3rd Ed.*) will be a complete revision of the 2002 edition. Check the National Resource Center Health and Safety in Child Care and Early Education website – http://nrckids.org – for updates.

EXECUTIVE SUMMARY

STANDARDS ON NUTRITION, PHYSICAL ACTIVITY, AND SCREEN TIME

Emerging research and evidence-based findings link children's eating nutritious food, engaging in daily age-appropriate physical activities, and limited screen time to maintaining a healthy weight. The reader can use this selected set of standards on nutrition, physical activity, and screen time in early care and education programs to build healthy lifestyles for generations to come. *Preventing Childhood Obesity in Early Care and Education Programs* is a targeted pre-release of a set of standards from *Caring for Our Children: National Health and Safety Performance Standards; Guidelines for Early Care and Education Programs, Third Edition* (*CFOC*)*. *CFOC*, the definitive source of published standards based on scientific evidence and expert consensus, supports key national campaigns for early development of healthy lifestyle habits such as *Let's Move* (1) and *Healthy Weight Initiative* (2), and is an unparalleled resource for creating model policies.

Teachers and caregivers are in a special position and are uniquely qualified to help children cultivate healthy eating and positive exercise habits that prevent childhood obesity. *CFOC* standards can assist early care and education programs, families, and community resources and agencies to develop and adopt safe and healthy practices, policies, and procedures that form a foundation of fitness for children that will last a lifetime.

Preventing Childhood Obesity in Early Care and Education Programs contains practical intervention strategies to prevent excessive weight gain in young children. The standards detail opportunities for facilities to work with families beginning on day one of an infant's enrollment, such as reaching out to mothers who breastfeed their infants by supporting them in a breastfeeding friendly environment.

CONTENTS

Preventing Childhood Obesity in Early Care and Education Programs presents a selected set of evidence-based and expert consensus-based standards in three topic areas: nutrition, physical activity, and screen time in early care and education.

- **Nutrition Standards**

  General Requirements: Feeding Plans; Use of USDA –CACFP Guidelines; Meal Pattern; Written Menus; Drinking Water and 100% Fruit Juice; Care of Children with Food Allergies, Vegetarian/Vegan Diets.

  Requirements for Infants: Breastfeeding; Feeding by a Consistent Caregiver/Teacher; Preparing, Feeding, Storing Human Milk or Formula; Techniques for Bottle Feeding; Introduction of Age-Appropriate Solid Food; Use of Soy-based Products.

  Requirements for Toddlers and Preschoolers: Meal and Snack Patterns; Serving Size, Encouraging Self-Feeding.

  Meal Service and Supervision: Socialization; Numbers of Children Fed Simultaneously by One Adult; Adult Supervision; Familiar and New Foods; Use of Nutritionist/Registered Dietitian.

  Food Brought from Home: Nutritional Quality of Food Brought from Home; Selection and Preparation of Food Brought from Home.

  Nutrition Education: Nutritional Learning Experiences for Children and Parents/Guardians; Health, Nutrition, Physical Activity, and Safety Awareness.

  Policies: Infant Feeding Policy; Food and Nutrition Service Policies and Plans.

- **Physical Activity Standards**

  Active Opportunities for Physical Activity and playtime (Outdoors and Indoors); Policies and Practices and Caregivers/Teachers' Encouragement of Physical Activity.

- **Screen Time Standard**

  Limiting Screen Time – Media, Computer Time.

SUGGESTED USES OF STANDARDS FOR PREVENTING CHILDHOOD OBESITY

- **Families** can join caregivers/teachers in planning programs to prevent childhood obesity and encourage healthy living. Families may also want to incorporate some of these same strategies and practices at home.
- **Caregivers/Teachers** can develop practices, policies, and staff training to ensure that children's programs include healthy, age-appropriate feeding, abundant physical activity, and limited screen time.
- **Health Care Professionals** are able to assist families and caregivers/teachers to choose feeding plans, develop active playtimes, and limit screen time that encourage children's development of healthy habits.
- **Regulators** have evidence-based rationale to develop regulations that support the prevention of obesity and promote healthy habits.
- **Early Childhood Systems** can build integrated nutrition and physical activity components into their systems that promote healthy lifestyles for all children.
- **Policy-makers** are equipped with sound science to meet emerging challenges to children's development of lifelong healthy behavior and life styles.
- **Academic Faculty** of early childhood education programs can instill healthy practices in their students to model and use with children upon entering the early childhood workplace.

PUBLISHERS: AAP, APHA, NRC

Collaborating on the development of health and safety best practices for children, the American Academy of Pediatrics (AAP), the American Public Health Association (APHA), and the National Resource Center for Health and Safety in Child Care and Early Education (NRC) publish *CFOC* (3rd edition to be released in 2011) with funding from the U.S. Department of Health and Human Services, Health Resources and Services Administration, Maternal and Child Health Bureau (MCHB). The long-lasting and positive relationship of AAP, APHA, NRC, and MCHB, a model of public-private partnership and inter-professional teamwork, has produced standards that meet the needs of many perspectives in the early childhood community.

1. The White House. 2010. *Let's move campaign.* http://www.letsmove.gov/
2. U.S. Department of Health and Human Services. 2010. *The Surgeon General's Vision for a Healthy and Fit Nation.* Rockville, MD: U.S. DHHS, OSG. http://www.surgeongeneral.gov/library/obesityvision/obesityvision2010.pdf.

**Caring for Our Children: National Health and Safety Performance Standards; Guidelines for Early Care Education Programs, Third Edition* (*CFOC 3rd Ed.*) will be a complete revision of the 2002 edition's 707 standards and appendices covering administration, child abuse, child development, children with special health care needs, environmental health, general health, infectious diseases, injury prevention, nutrition and physical activity, and staff health. Check the National Resource Center Health and Safety in Child Care and Early Education Website – http://nrckids.org – for updates.

NUTRITION STANDARDS

Introduction

One of the basic responsibilities of every parent/guardian and caregiver/teacher is to provide nourishing food daily that is clean, safe, and developmentally appropriate for children. Food is essential in any early care and education setting to keep infants and children free from hunger. Children also need freely available, clean drinking water. Feeding should occur in a relaxed and pleasant environment that fosters healthy digestion and positive social behavior. Food provides energy and nutrients needed by infants and children during the critical period of their growth and development.

Feeding nutritious food everyday must be accompanied by offering appropriate daily physical activity and play time for the healthy physical, social, and emotional development of infants and young children. There is solid evidence that physical activity can prevent a rapid gain in weight which leads to childhood obesity early in life. The early care and education setting is an ideal environment to foster the goal of providing supervised, age-appropriate physical activity during the critical years of growth when health habits and patterns are being developed for life. The overall benefits of practicing healthy eating patterns, while being physically active daily are significant. Physical, social, and emotional habits are developed during the early years and continue into adulthood; thus these habits can be improved in early childhood to prevent and reduce obesity and a range of chronic diseases. Active play and supervised structured physical activities promote healthy weight, improved overall fitness, including mental health, improved bone development, cardiovascular health, and development of social skills. The physical activity standards outline the blueprint for practical methods of achieving the goal of promoting healthy bodies and minds of young children.

Breastfeeding sets the stage for an infant to establish healthy attachment. The American Academy of Pediatrics, the United States Breastfeeding Committee, the Academy of Breastfeeding Medicine, the American Academy of Family Physicians, the World Health Organization, and the United Nations Children's Fund (UNICEF) all recommend that women should breastfeed exclusively for about the first six months of the infant's life, adding age-appropriate solid foods (complementary foods) and continuing breastfeeding for at least the first year if not longer.

Human milk, containing all the nutrients to promote optimal growth, is the most developmentally appropriate food for infants. It changes during the course of each feeding and over time to meet the growing child's changing nutritional needs. All caregivers/teachers should be trained to encourage, support, and advocate for breastfeeding. Caregivers/teachers have a unique opportunity to support breastfeeding mothers, who are often daunted by the prospect of continuing to breastfeed as they return to work. Early care and education programs can reduce a breastfeeding mother's anxiety by welcoming breastfeeding families and providing a staff that is well-trained in the proper handling of human milk and feeding of breastfed infants.

Mothers who formula feed can also establish healthy attachment. A mother may choose not to breastfeed her infant for reasons that may include: human milk is not available, there is a real or perceived inadequate supply of human milk, her infant fails to gain weight, there is an existing medical condition for which human milk is contraindicated, or a mother desires not to breastfeed. Today there is a range of infant formulas on the market that vary in nutrient content and address specific needs of individual infants. A primary care provider should prescribe the specific infant formula to be used to meet the nutritional requirements of an individual infant. When infant formula is used to supplement an infant being breastfed, the mother should be encouraged to continue to breastfeed or to pump human milk since her milk supply will decrease if her milk production isn't stimulated by breastfeeding or pumping.

Given adequate opportunity, assistance, and age-appropriate equipment, children learn to self-feed as age-appropriate solid foods are introduced. Equally important to self-feeding is children's attainment of normal physical growth, motor coordination, and cognitive and social skills. Modeling of healthy eating behavior by early care and education staff helps a child to develop lifelong healthy eating habits. This period, beginning at six months of age, is an opportune time for children to learn more about the world around them by expressing their independence. Children pick and choose from different kinds and combinations of foods offered. To ensure programs are offering a variety of foods, selections should be made from these groups of food:

Grains - especially whole grains;
Vegetables - dark, green leafy and deep yellow;
Fruits - deep orange, yellow, and red whole fruits, 100% fruit juices limited to no more than four to six ounces per day for children one year of age and over;
Milk - whole milk, or reduced fat (2%) milk for children at risk for obesity or hypercholesterolemia, for children from one year of age up to two years of age; skim or 1% for children two years or older, unsweetened low-fat yogurt or low-fat cheese (cottage, farmer's);
Meats and Beans - baked or broiled chicken, fish, lean meats, dried peas and beans; and
Oils - vegetable.

Current research supports a diet based on a variety of nutrient dense foods which provide substantial amounts of essential nutrients - protein, carbohydrates, oils, and vitamins and minerals - with appropriate calories to meet the child's needs. For children, the availability of a variety of clean, safe, nourishing foods is essential during a period of rapid growth and development. The nutrition and food service standards, along with related appendices, address age-appropriate foods and feeding techniques beginning with the very first food, preferably human milk and when not possible, infant formula based on the recommendation of the infant's primary care provider and family. As part of their developing growth and maturity, toddlers often exhibit changed eating habits compared to when they were infants. One may indulge in eating sprees, wanting to eat the same food for several days. Another may become a picky eater, picking or dawdling over food, or refusing to eat a certain food because it is new and unfamiliar with a new taste, color, odor, or texture. If these or other food behaviors persist, parents/guardians, caregivers/teachers, and the primary care provider together should determine the reason(s) and come up with a plan to address the issue. The consistency of the plan is important in helping a child to build sound eating habits during a time when they are focused on developing as an individual and often have erratic, unpredictable appetites. Family homes and center-based out-of-home early care and education settings have the opportunity to guide and support children's sound eating habits and food learning experiences (1-3).

Early food and eating experiences form the foundation of attitudes about food, eating behavior, and consequently, food habits. Responsive feeding, where the parents/guardians or caregivers/teachers recognize and respond to infant and child cues, helps foster trust and reduces overfeeding. Sound food habits are built on eating and enjoying a variety of healthful foods. Including culturally specific family foods is a dietary goal for feeding infants and young children. Current research documents that a balanced diet, combined with daily and routine age-appropriate physical activity, can reduce diet-related risks of overweight, obesity, and chronic disease later in life (1). Two essentials - eating healthy foods and engaging in physical activity on a daily basis - promote a healthy beginning during the early years and throughout the life span. *Dietary Guidelines for Americans, 2005* and *My Pyramid for Kids* are designed to support lifestyle behaviors that promote health, including a diet composed of a variety of healthy foods and physical activity at two years of age and older (4-7).

REFERENCES:
1. U.S. Department of Health and Human Services, U.S. Department of Agriculture. 2005. *Dietary guidelines for Americans, 2005*. 6th ed. Washington, DC: U.S. Government Printing Office. http://www.health.gov/dietaryguidelines/dga2005/document/pdf/DGA2005.pdf.
2. U.S. Department of Agriculture. 2010. *MyPyramid*. http://www.mypyramid.gov.
3. Zero to Three. 2007. *Healthy from the start—How feeding nurtures your young child's body, heart, and mind*. Washington, DC: Zero to Three.
4. Pipes, P. L., C. M. Trahms, eds. 1997. *Nutrition in infancy and childhood*. 6th ed. New York: McGraw-Hill.
5. Marotz, L. R. 2008. *Health, safety, and nutrition for the young child*. 7th ed. Clifton Park, NY: Delmar Learning.
6. Herr, J. 2008. *Working with young children*. 4th ed. Tinley Park, IL: Goodheart-Willcox Company.
7. Dalton, S. 2004. *Our overweight children: What parents, schools, and communities can do to control the fatness epidemic*. Berkeley, CA: University of California Press.

General Requirements

Written Nutrition Plan

STANDARD: The facility should provide nourishing and attractive food for children according to a written plan developed by a qualified Nutritionist/Registered Dietitian. Caregivers/teachers, directors, and food service personnel should share the responsibility for carrying out the plan. The administrator is responsible for implementing the plan but may delegate tasks to caregivers/teachers and food service personnel. Where infants and young children are involved, special attention to the feeding plan may include attention to supporting mothers in maintaining their human milk supply. The nutrition plan should include steps to take when problems require rapid response by the staff, such as when a child chokes during mealtime or has an allergic reaction to a food. The completed plan should be on file, easily accessible to staff, and available to parents/guardians upon request.

If the facility is large enough to justify employment of a full-time Nutritionist/Registered Dietitian or Child Care Food Service Manager, the facility should delegate to this person the responsibility for implementing the written plan.

Some children may have medical conditions that require special dietary modifications. A written care plan from the primary care provider, clearly stating the food(s) to be avoided and food(s) to be substituted should be on file. This information should be updated periodically if the modification is not a lifetime special dietary need. Staff should be trained about a child's dietary modification to ensure that no child in care ingests inappropriate foods while at the facility. The proper modifications should be implemented whether the child brings their own food or whether it is prepared on site. The facility needs to inform all families and staff if certain foods, such as nut products (example: peanut butter), should not be brought from home because of a child's life-threatening allergy. Staff should also know what procedure to follow if ingestion occurs. In addition to knowing ahead of time what procedures to follow, staff must know their designated roles during an emergency. The emergency plan should be dated and updated.

RATIONALE: Nourishing and attractive food is the cornerstone for children's health, growth, and development as well as developmentally appropriate learning experiences (1-9). Nutrition and feeding are fundamental and required in every facility. Because children grow and develop more rapidly during the first few years of life than at any other time, the child's home and the facility together must provide food that is adequate in amount and type to meet each child's growth and nutritional needs. Children can learn healthy eating habits and be better equipped to maintain a healthy weight if they eat nourishing food while attending early care and education settings and if they are allowed to feed themselves and determine the amount of food they will ingest at any one sitting. The obesity epidemic makes this an important lesson today.

Meals and snacks provide the caregiver/teacher an opportunity to model appropriate mealtime behavior and guide the conversation, which aids in children's conceptual, sensory language development and eye/hand coordination. In larger facilities, professional nutrition staff must be involved to assure compliance with nutrition and food service guidelines, including accommodation of children with special health care needs.

COMMENTS: *Making Food Healthy and Safe for Children, 2nd Ed.* (http://nti.unc.edu/course_files/curriculum/nutrition/making_food_healthy_and_safe.pdf) contains practical tips for implementing the standards for culturally diverse groups of infants and children.

RELATED STANDARDS:

Assessment and Planning of Nutrition for Individual Children
Feeding Plans and Dietary Modifications
Use of Nutritionist/Registered Dietitian
Nutrition Learning Experiences for Children
Food and Nutrition Service Policies and Plans
Appendix - Nutritionists, Registered Dietitian, Consultant, and Food Services Staff

REFERENCES:

1. U.S. Department of Health and Human Services, Administration for Children and Families, Office of Head Start. 2009. *Head Start program performance standards*. Rev. ed. Washington, DC: U.S. Government Printing Office. http://eclkc.ohs.acf.hhs.gov/hslc/Program%20Design%20and%20Management/Head%20Start%20Requirements/Head%20Start%20Requirements/45%20CFR%20Chapter%20XIII/45%20CFR%20Chap%20XIII_ENG.pdf.
2. Hagan, J. F., J. S. Shaw, P. M. Duncan, eds. 2008. *Bright futures: Guidelines for health supervision of infants, children, and adolescents*. 3rd ed. Elk Grove Village, IL: American Academy of Pediatrics.
3. Story, M., K. Holt, D. Sofka, eds. 2002. *Bright futures in practice: Nutrition*. 2nd ed. Arlington, VA: National Center for Education in Maternal and Child Health. http://www.brightfutures.org/nutrition/pdf/frnt_mttr.pdf.
4. Wardle, F., N. Winegarner. 1992. Nutrition and Head Start. *Child Today* 21:57.
5. Benjamin, S. E., ed. 2007. *Making food healthy and safe for children: How to meet the national health and safety performance standards – Guidelines for out of home child care programs*. 2nd ed. Chapel Hill, NC: National Training Institute for Child Care Health Consultants. http://nti.unc.edu/course_files/curriculum/nutrition/making_food_healthy_and_safe.pdf
6. Dietz, W. H., L. Stern, eds. 1998. *American Academy of Pediatrics guide to your child's nutrition*. New York: Villard.
7. Kleinman, R. E., ed. 2009. *Pediatric nutrition handbook*. 6th ed. Elk Grove Village, IL: American Academy of Pediatrics.
8. Lally, J. R., A. Griffin, E. Fenichel, M. Segal, E. Szanton, B. Weissbourd. 2003. *Caring for infants and toddlers in groups: Developmentally appropriate practice*. Arlington, VA: Zero to Three.
9. Enders, J. B., R. E. Rockwell. 2003. *Food, nutrition, and the young child*. 4th ed. New York: Macmillan.

Routine Health Supervision and Growth Monitoring

STANDARD: The facility should require that each child has routine health supervision by the child's primary care provider, according to the standards of the American Academy of Pediatrics (AAP) (3). For all children, health supervision includes routine screening tests, immunizations, and chronic or acute illness monitoring. For children younger than twenty-four months of age, health supervision includes documentation and plotting of charts on standard sex-specific length, weight, weight for length, and head circumference and assessing diet and activity. For children twenty-four months of age and older, sex-specific height and weight graphs should be plotted by the primary care provider in addition to body mass index (BMI). BMI is classified as underweight (less than 5%), healthy weight (BMI 5%-84%), overweight (BMI 85%-94%), and obese (BMI equal to or greater than 95%). Follow up visits with the child's primary care provider that include a full assessment and laboratory evaluations should be scheduled for children with weight for length greater than 95% and BMI greater than 85%.

School health services can meet this standard for school-age children in care if they meet the AAP's standards for school-age children and if the results of each child's examinations are shared with the caregiver/teacher as well as with the school health system. With parental/guardian consent, pertinent health information should be exchanged among the child's routine source of health care and all participants in the child's care, including any school health program involved in the care of the child.

RATIONALE: Provision of routine preventive health services for children ensures healthy growth and development and helps detect disease when it is most treatable. Immunization prevents or reduces diseases for which effective vaccines are available. When children are receiving care that involves the school health system, such care should be coordinated by the exchange of information, with parental/guardian permission, among the school health system, the child's medical home, and the caregiver/teacher. Such exchange will ensure that all participants in the child's care are aware of the child's health status and follow a common care plan.

The plotting of height and weight measurements and plotting and classification of BMI (Body Mass Index) by the primary care provider or school health personnel, on a reference growth chart, will show how children are growing over time and how they compare with other children of the same chronological age and sex (1,3,4). Growth charts are based on data from national probability samples, representative of children in the general population. Their use by the primary care provider may facilitate early recognition of growth concerns, leading to further evaluation, diagnosis, and the development of a plan of care. Such a plan of care, if communicated to the caregiver/teacher, can direct the caregiver/teacher's attention to disease, poor nutrition, or inadequate physical activity that requires modification of feeding or other health practices in the early care and education setting (2).

COMMENTS: Periodic and accurate height and weight measurements that are obtained, plotted, and interpreted by a person who is competent in performing these tasks provide an important indicator of health status. If such measurements are made in the early care and education facility, the data from the measurements should be shared by the facility, subject to parental/guardian consent, with everyone involved in the child's care, including parents/guardians, caregivers/teachers, and the child's primary care provider. The Child Care Health Consultant can provide staff training on growth assessment. It is important to maintain strong linkage among the early care and education facility, school, parent/guardian, and the child's primary care provider. Screening results (physical and behavioral) and laboratory assessments are only useful if a plan for care can be developed to initiate and maintain lifestyle changes that incorporate the child's activities during their time at the early care and education program.

The Special Supplemental Nutrition Program for Women, Infants, and Children (WIC) can also be a source for the BMI data with parental/guardian consent, as WIC tracks growth and development if the child is enrolled.

For BMI charts by sex and age, see http://www.cdc.gov/growthcharts/clinical_charts.htm.

RELATED STANDARDS:

Assessment and Planning of Nutrition for Individual Children

REFERENCES:

1. Paige, D. M. 1988. *Clinical nutrition*. 2nd ed. St. Louis: Mosby.
2. Kleinman, R. E. 2009. *Pediatric nutrition handbook*. 6th ed. Elk Grove Village, IL: American Academy of Pediatrics.
3. Hagan, J. F., J. S. Shaw, P. M. Duncan. 2008. *Bright futures: Guidelines for health supervision of infants, children, and adolescents*. 3rd ed. Elk Grove Village, IL: American Academy of Pediatrics.
4. Story, M., K. Holt, D. Sofka, eds. 2002. *Bright futures in practice: Nutrition*. 2nd ed. Arlington, VA: National Center for Education in Maternal and Child Health. http://www.brightfutures.org/nutrition/pdf/frnt_mttr.pdf.

Assessment and Planning of Nutrition for Individual Children

STANDARD: As a part of routine health supervision by the child's primary care provider, children should be evaluated for nutrition-related medical problems such as failure to thrive, overweight, obesity, food allergy, reflux disease, and iron-deficiency anemia. The nutritional standards throughout this document are general recommendations that may not always be appropriate for some children with medically-identified special nutrition needs. Caregivers/teachers should communicate with the child's parent/guardian and primary care provider to adapt nutritional offerings to individual children as indicated and medically-appropriate. Caregivers/teachers should work with the parent/guardian to implement individualized feeding plans developed by the child's primary care provider to meet a child's unique nutritional needs. These plans could include, for instance, additional iron-rich foods to a child who has been diagnosed as having iron-deficiency anemia. For a child diagnosed as overweight, the plan would focus on controlling portion sizes. Also calorie dense foods like sugar sweetened juices, nectars, and beverages should not be served. Denying a child food that others are eating is difficult to explain and difficult for some children to understand and accept. Attention should be paid to teaching about proper portion sizes and the average daily caloric intake of the child.

Some children require special feeding techniques such as thickened foods or special positioning during meals. Other children will require dietary modifications based on food intolerances such as lactose or wheat (gluten) intolerance. Some children will need dietary modifications based on cultural or religious preferences such as vegetarian or kosher diets.

RATIONALE: The early years are a critical time for children's growth and development. Nutritional problems must be identified and treated during this period in order to prevent serious or long-term medical problems. The early care and education setting may be offering a majority of a child's daily nutritional intake especially for children in full-time care. It is important that the facility ensures that food offerings are congruent with nutritional interventions or dietary modifications recommended by the child's primary care provider in consultation with the Nutritionist/Registered Dietitian to make certain that intervention is child specific.

RELATED STANDARDS

Routine Health Supervision and Growth Monitoring
Feeding Plans and Dietary Modifications

Feeding Plans and Dietary Modifications

STANDARD: Before a child enters an early care and education facility, the facility should obtain a written history that contains any special nutrition or feeding needs for the child, including use of human milk or any special feeding utensils. The staff should review this history with the child's parents/guardians, clarifying and discussing how parental home feeding routines may differ from the facility's planned routine. The child's primary care provider should provide written information about any dietary modifications or special feeding techniques that are required at the early care and education program and these plans should be shared with the child's parents/guardians upon request.

If dietary modifications are indicated, based on a child's medical or special dietary needs, the caregiver/teacher should modify or supplement the child's diet to meet the individual child's specific needs. Dietary modifications should be made in consultation with the parents/guardians and the child's primary care provider. Caregivers/teachers can consult with a Nutritionist/Registered Dietitian.

Reasons for modification of a child's diet may be related to food sensitivity. Food sensitivity includes a range of conditions in which a child exhibits an adverse reaction to a food that, in some instances, can be life threatening. Modification of a child's diet may be related to a food allergy, inability to digest or to tolerate certain foods, need for extra calories, need for special positioning while eating, diabetes and the need to match food with insulin, food idiosyncrasies, and other identified feeding issues. Examples include celiac disease, phenylketonuria, diabetes, severe food allergy (anaphylaxis), and others. In some cases, a child may become ill if the child is unable to eat, so missing a meal could have a negative consequence, especially for diabetics.

For a child identified with special health care needs for dietary modification or special feeding techniques, written instructions from the child's parent/guardian and the child's primary care provider should be provided in the child's record and carried out accordingly. Dietary modifications should be recorded. These written instructions must identify:

a) The child's full name and date of instructions;
b) The child's special needs;
c) Any dietary restrictions based on the special needs;
d) Any special feeding or eating utensils;
e) Any foods to be omitted from the diet and any foods to be substituted;
f) Limitations of life activities;
g) Any other pertinent special needs information;
h) What, if anything, needs to be done if the child is exposed to restricted foods.

The written history of special nutrition or feeding needs should be used to develop individual feeding plans and, collectively, to develop facility menus. Disciplines related to special nutrition needs, including nutrition, nursing, speech, occupational therapy and physical therapy, should participate when needed and/or when they are available to the facility. The Nutritionist/Registered Dietitian should approve menus that accommodate needed dietary modifications.

The feeding plan should include steps to take when a situation arises that requires rapid response by the staff, such as a child's choking during mealtime or a child with a known history of food allergies demonstrating signs and symptoms of anaphylaxis (severe allergic reaction, e.g., difficulty breathing or severe redness and swelling of the face or mouth). The completed plan should be on file and accessible to the staff and available to parents/guardians upon request.

RATIONALE: Children with special health care needs may have individual requirements related to diet and swallowing, involving special feeding utensils and feeding needs that will necessitate the development of an individual plan prior to their entry into the facility (1-3). A number of children with special health care needs have difficulty with feeding, including delayed attainment of basic chewing, swallowing, and independent feeding skills. Food, eating style, food utensils, and equipment, including furniture, may have to be adapted to meet the developmental and physical needs of individual children (1-3).

Some children have difficulty with slow weight gain and need their caloric intake monitored and supplemented. Others with special needs, such as those with diabetes, may need to have their diet matched to their medication (insulin if they are on a fixed dose of insulin). Some children are unable to tolerate certain foods because of their allergy to the food or their inability to digest it. In children, foods are the most common cause of anaphylaxis. Nuts, seeds, eggs, soy, milk, and seafood are among the most common allergens for food-induced anaphylaxis in children (3). Staff members must know ahead of time what procedures to follow, as well as their designated roles during an emergency.

As a safety and health precaution, the staff should know in advance whether a child has food allergies, inborn errors of metabolism, diabetes, celiac disease, tongue thrust, or special health care needs related to feeding, such as requiring special feeding utensils or equipment, nasogastric or gastric tube feedings, or special positioning. These situations require individual planning prior to the child's entry into early care and education and on an ongoing basis (3,4).

In some cases, dietary modifications are based on religious or cultural beliefs. Detailed information on each child's special needs whether stemming from dietary, feeding equipment, or cultural needs, is invaluable to the facility staff in meeting the nutritional needs of that child.

COMMENTS: Close collaboration between the home and the facility is necessary for children on special diets. Parents/guardians may have to provide food on a temporary or, even, a permanent basis, if the facility, after exploring all community resources, is unable to provide the special diet.

RELATED STANDARDS:
Assessment and Planning of Nutrition for Individual Children

REFERENCES:
1. Samour, P. Q., K. King. 2005. *Handbook of pediatric nutrition*. 3rd ed. Lake Dallas, TX: Helm.
2. Dietz, W. H., L. Stern, eds. 1998. *American Academy of Pediatrics guide to your child's nutrition*. New York: Villard.
3. Kleinman, R. E., ed. 2009. *Pediatric nutrition handbook*. 6th ed. Elk Grove Village, IL: American Academy of Pediatrics.
4. Lally, J. R., A. Griffin, E. Fenichel, M. Segal, E. Szanton, B. Weissbourd. 2003. *Caring for infants and toddlers in groups: Developmentally appropriate practice*. Arlington, VA: Zero to Three.

Use of USDA - CACFP Guidelines

STANDARD: All meals and snacks and their preparation, service, and storage should meet the requirements for meals of the child care component of the U.S. Department of Agriculture (USDA), Child and Adult Care Food Program (CACFP), and the 7 Code of Federal Regulations (CFR) Part 226.20 (1,5).

RATIONALE: The CACFP regulations, policies, and guidance materials on meal requirements provide the basic guidelines for sound nutrition and sanitation practices. Meals and snacks offered to young children should provide a variety of nourishing foods on a frequent basis to meet the nutritional needs of infants from birth to children age twelve (2-4). The CACFP guidance for meals and snack patterns ensures that the nutritional needs of infants and children, including school-age children up through age twelve, are met based on current scientific knowledge (5). Programs not eligible for reimbursement under the regulations of CACFP should use the CACFP food guidance.

COMMENTS: The staff should use information on the child's growth in developing individual feeding plans. For the current CACFP meal patterns, go to http://www.fns.usda.gov/cnd/care/ProgramBasics/Meals/Meal_Patterns.htm.

RELATED STANDARDS:

Routine Health Supervision and Growth Monitoring
Categories of Foods
Meal and Snack Patterns
Meal and Snack Patterns for Toddlers and Preschoolers
Meal and Snack Patterns for School-age Children

REFERENCES:

1. Lally, J. R., A. Griffin, E. Fenichel, M. Segal, E. Szanton, B. Weissbourd. 2003. *Caring for infants and toddlers in groups: Developmentally appropriate practice*. Arlington, VA: Zero to Three.
2. U.S. Department of Agriculture, Child and Adult Care Food Program. 2002. *Menu magic for children: A menu planning guide for child care*. Washington, DC: USDA, FNS. http://www.fns.usda.gov/tn/resources/menu_magic.pdf.
3. U.S. Department of Agriculture, Team Nutrition. 2000. *Building blocks for fun and healthy meals: A menu planner for the child and adult care food program*. Washington, DC: USDA, Food and Nutrition Service. http://teamnutrition.usda.gov/Resources/blocksintro.pdf.
4. U.S. Department of Agriculture, Team Nutrition. 2010. Child care providers: Healthy meals resource system. http://healthymeals.nal.usda.gov/nal_display/index.php?tax_level=1&info_center=14&tax_subject=264.
5. U.S. Department of Agriculture, Food and Nutrition Service. 2010. Child and Adult Care Food Program (CACFP). http://www.fns.usda.gov/cnd/care/.

Categories of Foods

STANDARD: Children in care should be offered items of food from the following categories:

Making Healthy Food Choices		
Food Groups	**USDA***	**Guidelines for Young Children**
Grains	Grains & Breads: Make 1/2 your grains whole	Whole Grains - breads, cereals, pastas
Vegetables	Vegetables & Fruits: Vary your veggies	· Dark green, orange, deep yellow vegetables · Other vegetables including potatoes, other root vegetables, such as viandas
Fruits	Vegetables & Fruits: Focus on fruits	· Eat a variety, especially whole fruits · Whole fruit, mashed or pureed, for infants 7 months up to one year of age · No juice before 12 months of age · 4 to 6 oz juice /day for 1 to 6 year olds · 8 to 12 oz juice/day for 7 to 12 year olds
Milk	Milk: Get your calcium-rich foods	· Human milk, infant formula · Whole milk for children ages 1 year of age up to 2 years of age or reduced fat (2%) milk for those at risk for obesity or hypercholesterolemia · 1% or skim milk for children 2 years of age and older · Other milk equivalent products such as yogurt and cottage cheese (low-fat for children 2 years of age and older)
Meat & Beans	Meat & Meat Alternatives: Go lean with protein	· Chicken, fish, lean meat · Legumes (dried peas, beans) · Avoid fried meats
Oils	Know the limits on fats	· Choose monounsaturated and polyunsaturated fats (olive oil, safflower oil) · Avoid trans fats, saturated fats and fried foods
Sugar/salt	Know the limits of sugars and salt (sodium)	Avoid or Limit: · Avoid concentrated sweets such as candy, sodas, sweetened drinks, fruit nectars, and flavored milk · Limit salty foods such as chips and pretzels

*Recommends: Find your balance between food and physical activity

Additional Resources:

U.S. Department of Health and Human Services. 2010. *The Surgeon General's vision for a healthy and fit nation*. Rockville, MD: U.S. DHHS. OSG. http://www.surgeongeneral.gov/library/obesityvision/obesityvision2010.pdf.

U.S. Department of Health and Human Services, U.S. Department of Agriculture. 2005. *Dietary guidelines for Americans, 2005*. 6th ed. Washington, DC: U.S. Government Printing Office. http://www.health.gov/dietaryguidelines/dga2005/document/pdf/DGA2005.pdf.

U.S. Department of Health and Human Services, Office of Disease Prevention and Health Promotion. 2008. *2008 physical activity guidelines for Americans*. Rockville, MD: U.S. Government Printing Office. http://www.health.gov/paguidelines/guidelines/default.aspx.

Story, M., K. Holt, D. Sofka, eds. 2002. *Bright futures in practice: Nutrition*. 2nd ed. Arlington, VA: National Center for Education in Maternal and Child Health. http://www.brightfutures.org/nutrition/pdf/frnt_mttr.pdf.

U.S. Department of Agriculture. 2008. *MyPyramid for Kids*. www.mypyramid.gov.

RATIONALE: Both the *Dietary Guidelines for Americans, 2005* and the U.S. Department of Agriculture (USDA) identify and suggest use of food groups as a basis for making wise choices of nutritious foods from each of the five food groups (1-3). Using the food groups as a tool is a practical approach to select foods high in essential nutrients and moderate in calories/energy. Meals and snacks planned based on the five food groups promote normal growth and development of children as well as reduce their risk of overweight, obesity and related chronic diseases later in life. Age-specific guidance for meals and snacks is outlined in CACFP guidelines and accessible at http://www.fns.usda.gov/cnd/care/ProgramBasics/Meals/Meal_Patterns.htm. Early care and education settings provide the opportunity for children to learn about the food they eat, to develop and strengthen their fine and gross motor skills, and to engage in social interaction at mealtimes.

COMMENTS: For more information on portion sizes and types of food, see CACFP Guidelines at http://www.fns.usda.gov/cnd/care/ProgramBasics/Meals/Meal_Patterns.htm.

RELATED STANDARDS

Feeding Plans and Dietary Modifications
Meal and Snack Patterns
100% Fruit Juice
Meal and Snack Patterns for Toddlers and Preschoolers
Meal and Snack Patterns for School-Age Children
Preparing, Feeding, and Storing Human Milk
Preparing, Feeding, and Storing Infant Formula
Feeding Cow's Milk
Nutritional Learning Experiences for Children
Nutrition Education for Parents/Guardians
Appendix - MyPyramid for Preschoolers Mini-Poster
Appendix - MyPyramid for Kids Poster

REFERENCES:

1. U.S. Department of Health and Human Services, U.S. Department of Agriculture. 2005. *Dietary guidelines for Americans, 2005.* 6th ed. Washington, DC: U.S. Government Printing Office. http://www.health.gov/dietaryguidelines/dga2005/document/pdf/DGA2005.pdf.
2. U.S. Department of Agriculture, Food and Nutrition Service. 2010. Child and adult care food program (CACFP). http://www.fns.usda.gov/cnd/care/.
3. Nemours Health and Prevention Services. 2008. *Best practices for healthy eating: A guide to help children grow up healthy.* Version 2. Newark, DE: Nemours Foundation. http://www.nemours.org/content/dam/nemours/www/filebox/service/preventive/nhps/heguide.pdf

Meal and Snack Patterns

STANDARD: The facility should ensure that the following meal and snack pattern occurs:

a) Children in care for eight and fewer hours in one day should be offered at least one meal and two snacks or two meals and one snack.

b) Children in care more than eight hours in one day should be offered at least two meals and two snacks or three snacks and one meal.

c) A nutritious snack should be offered to all children in midmorning (if they are not offered a breakfast on-site that is provided within three hours of lunch) and in the middle of the afternoon.

d) Children should be offered food at intervals at least two hours apart and not more than three hours apart unless the child is asleep. Some very young infants may need to be fed at shorter intervals than every two hours to meet their nutritional needs, especially breastfed infants being fed expressed human milk. Lunch service may need to be served to toddlers earlier than the preschool-aged children due to their need for an earlier nap schedule. Children must be awake prior to being offered a meal/snack.

e) Children should be allowed time to eat their food and not be rushed during the meal or snack service. They should not be allowed to play during these times.

f) Caregivers/teachers should discuss the breastfed infant's feeding patterns with the parents/guardians because the frequency of breastfeeding at home can vary. For example, some infants may still be feeding frequently at night, while others may do the bulk of their feeding during the day. Knowledge about the infant's feeding patterns over twenty-four hours will help caregivers/teachers assess the infant's feeding during his/her time with the caregiver/teacher.

RATIONALE: Young children, under the age of six, need to be offered food every two to three hours. Appetite and interest in food varies from one meal or snack to the next. To ensure that the child's daily nutritional needs are met, small feedings of nourishing food should be scheduled over the course of a day (1-6). Snacks should be nutritious, as they often are a significant part of a child's daily intake. Children in care for more than eight hours need additional food because this period represents a majority of a young child's waking hours.

COMMENTS: Caloric needs vary greatly from one child to another. A child may require more food during growth spurts. Some states have regulations indicating suggested times for meals and snacks. By regulation, in the Child and Adult Care Food Program (CACFP), centers and family child care homes may be approved to claim up to two reimbursable meals (breakfast, lunch or supper) and one snack, or two snacks and one meal, for each eligible participant, each day. Many after-school programs provide before school care or full day care when elementary school is out of session. Many of these programs offer either a breakfast and/or a morning snack. After-school care programs may claim reimbursement for serving each child one snack, each day. In some states after-school programs also have the option of providing a supper. These are reimbursed by CACFP if they meet certain guidelines and timeframes. For more information on CACFP meal reimbursement see the CACFP Website - http://www.fns.usda.gov/cnd/care/CACFP/aboutcacfp.htm.

RELATED STANDARDS:

Meal and Snack Patterns for Toddlers and Preschoolers
Meal and Snack Patterns for School-Age Children

REFERENCES:

1. U.S. Department of Health and Human Services, Administration for Children and Families, Office of Head Start. 2009. *Head Start program performance standards*. Rev. ed. Washington, DC: U.S. Government Printing Office. http://eclkc.ohs.acf.hhs.gov/hslc/Program%20Design%20and%20Management/Head%20Start%20Requirements/Head%20Start%20Requirements/45%20CFR%20Chapter%20XIII/45%20CFR%20Chap%20XIII_ENG.pdf.
2. Benjamin, S. E., ed. 2007. *Making food healthy and safe for children: How to meet the national health and safety performance standards – Guidelines for out of home child care programs*. 2nd ed. Chapel Hill, NC: National Training Institute for Child Care Health Consultants. http://nti.unc.edu/course_files/curriculum/nutrition/making_food_healthy_and_safe.pdf.
3. Pipes, P. L., C. M. Trahms, eds. 1997. *Nutrition in infancy and childhood*. 6th ed. New York: McGraw-Hill.
4. Butte, N., S. K. Cobb. 2004. The Start Healthy feeding guidelines for infants and children. *J Am Diet Assoc* 104:442-54.
5. Kleinman, R. E., ed. 2009. *Pediatric nutrition handbook*. 6th ed. Elk Grove Village, IL: American Academy of Pediatrics.
6. Plemas, C., B. M. Popkin. 2010. Trends in snacking among U.S. children. *Health Affairs* 29:399-404.

Availability of Drinking Water

STANDARD: Clean, sanitary drinking water should be readily available, in indoor and outdoor areas, throughout the day. Water should not be a substitute for milk at meals or snacks where milk is a required food component unless it is recommended by the child's primary care provider.

On hot days, infants receiving human milk in a bottle can be given additional human milk in a bottle but should not be given water, especially in the first six months of life. Infants receiving formula and water can be given additional formula in a bottle. Toddlers and older children will need additional water as physical activity and/or hot temperatures cause their needs to increase. Children should learn to drink water from a cup or drinking fountain without mouthing the fixture. They should not be allowed to have water continuously in hand in a "sippy cup" or bottle. Permitting toddlers to suck continuously on a bottle or sippy cup filled with water, in order to soothe themselves, may cause nutritional or in rare instances, electrolyte imbalances. When tooth brushing is not done after a feeding, children should be offered water to drink to rinse food from their teeth.

RATIONALE: When children are thirsty between meals and snacks, water is the best choice. Encouraging children to learn to drink water in place of fruit drinks, soda, fruit nectars, or other sweetened drinks builds a beneficial habit. Drinking water during the day can reduce the extra caloric intake which is associated with overweight and obesity (1). Drinking water is good for a child's hydration and reduces acid in the mouth that contributes to early childhood caries (1,3,4). Water needs vary among young children and increase during times in which dehydration is a risk (e.g., hot summer days, during exercise, and in dry days in winter) (2).

COMMENTS: Clean, small pitchers of water and single-use paper cups available in the classrooms and on the playgrounds allow children to serve themselves water when they are thirsty. Drinking fountains should be kept clean and sanitary and maintained to provide adequate drainage.

RELATED STANDARDS:

Preparing, Feeding, and Storing Human Milk
Preparing, Feeding, and Storing Infant Formula
Playing Outdoors

REFERENCES:

1. Kleinman, R. E., ed. 2009. *Pediatric nutrition handbook*. 6th ed. Elk Grove

Village, IL: American Academy of Pediatrics.
2. Manz, F. 2007. Hydration in children. *J Am Coll Nutr* 26:562S-569S.
3. Casamassimo, P., K. Holt, eds. 2004. *Bright futures in practice: Oral health–pocket guide*. Washington, DC: National Maternal and Child Oral Health Resource Center. http://www.mchoralhealth.org/PDFs/BFOHPocketGuide.pdf.
4. Centers for Disease Control and Prevention. 2010. Community water fluoridation: Frequently asked questions. http://www.cdc.gov/fluoridation/faqs.htm.

100% Fruit Juice

STANDARD: The facility should serve only full-strength (100%) pasteurized fruit juice or full-strength fruit juice diluted with water from a cup to children twelve months of age or older. Juice should have no added sweeteners. The facility should offer juice at specific meals and snacks instead of continuously throughout the day. Juice consumption should be no more than a total of four to six ounces a day for children aged one to six years. This amount includes juice served at home. Children ages seven through twelve years of age should consume no more than a total of eight to twelve ounces of fruit juice per day. Caregivers/teachers should ask parents/guardians if they provide juice at home and how much. This information is important to know if and when to serve juice. Infants should not be given any fruit juice before twelve months of age. Whole fruit, mashed or pureed, is recommended for infants seven months up to one year of age.

RATIONALE: Whole fruit is more nutritious than fruit juice and provides dietary fiber. Fruit juice which is 100% offers no nutritional advantage over whole fruits.

Limiting the feeding of juice to specific meals and snacks will reduce acids produced by bacteria in the mouth that cause tooth decay. The frequency of exposure, rather than the quantity of food, is important in determining whether foods cause tooth decay. Although sugar is not the only dietary factor likely to cause tooth decay, it is a major factor in the prevalence of tooth decay (1,2).

Drinks that are called fruit juice drinks, fruit punches, or fruit nectars contain less than 100% fruit juice and are of a lower nutritional value than 100% fruit juice. Liquids with high sugar content have no place in a healthy diet and should be avoided. Continuous consumption of juice during the day has been associated with a decrease in appetite for other nutritious foods which can result in feeding problems and overweight/obesity. Infants should not be given juice from bottles or easily transportable, covered cups (e.g. sippy cups) that allow them to consume juice throughout the day.

The American Academy of Pediatrics (AAP) recommends that children aged one to six years drink no more than four to six ounces of fruit juice a day (3). This amount is the total quantity for the whole day, including both time at early care and education and at home. Caregivers/teachers should not give the entire amount while a child is in their care. For breastfed infants, AAP recommends that gradual introduction of iron-fortified foods may occur no sooner than around four months, but preferably six months to complement the human milk. Infants should not be given juice before they reach twelve months of age.

Overconsumption of 100% fruit juice can contribute to overweight and obesity (3-6). One study found that two- to five-year-old children who drank twelve or more ounces of fruit juice a day were more likely to be obese than those who drank less juice (2). Excessive fruit juice consumption may be associated with malnutrition (over nutrition and under nutrition), diarrhea, flatulence, and abdominal distention (3). Unpasteurized fruit juice may contain pathogens that can cause serious illnesses (3). The U.S. Food and Drug Administration requires a warning on the dangers of harmful bacteria on all unpasteurized juice or products (7).

COMMENTS: Caregivers/teachers, as well as many parents/guardians, should strive to understand the relationship between the consumption of sweetened beverages and tooth decay. Drinks with high sugar content should be avoided because they can contribute to childhood obesity (2,5,6), tooth decay, and poor nutrition.

RELATED STANDARDS:
Categories of Food

REFERENCES:
1. Casamassimo, P., K. Holt, eds. 2004. *Bright futures in practice: Oral health–pocket guide*. Washington, DC: National Maternal and Child Oral Health Resource Center. http://www.mchoralhealth.org/PDFs/BFOHPocketGuide.pdf.
2. Dennison, B. A., H. L. Rockwell, S. L. Baker. 1997. Excess fruit juice consumption by preschool-aged children is associated with short stature and obesity. *Pediatrics* 99:15-22.
3. American Academy of Pediatrics, Committee on Nutrition. 2007. Policy statement: The use and misuse of fruit juice in pediatrics. *Pediatrics* 119:405.
4. Faith, M. S., B. A. Dennison, L. S. Edmunds, H. H. Stratton. 2006. Fruit juice intake predicts increased adiposity gain in children from low-income families: Weight status-by-environment interaction. *Pediatrics* 118:2066-75.
5. Dubois, L., A. Farmer, M. Girard, K. Peterson. 2007. Regular sugar-sweetened beverage consumption between meals increases risk of overweight among preschool-aged children. *J Am Diet Assoc* 107:924-34.

6. Dennison, B. A., H. L. Rockwell, M. J. Nichols, P. Jenkins. 1999. Children's growth parameters vary by type of fruit juice consumed. *J Am Coll Nutr* 18:346-52.
7. U.S. Food and Drug Administration. *Safe handling of raw produce and fresh-squeezed fruit and vegetable juices*. New York: JMH Education. http://www.fda.gov/Food/ResourcesForYou/Consumers/ucm114299.htm.

Written Menus and Introduction of New Foods

STANDARD: Facilities should develop, at least one month in advance, written menus showing all foods to be served during that month and should make the menus available to parents/guardians. The facility should date and retain these menus for six months, unless the state regulatory agency requires a longer retention time. The menus should be amended to reflect any and all changes in the food actually served. Any substitutions should be of equal nutrient value.

To avoid problems of food sensitivity in very young children under eighteen months of age, caregivers/teachers should obtain from the child's parents/guardians a list of foods that have already been introduced (without any reaction), and then serve some of these foods to the child. As new foods are considered for serving, caregivers/teachers should share and discuss these foods with the parents/guardians prior to their introduction.

RATIONALE: Planning menus in advance helps to ensure that food will be on hand. Parents/guardians need to be informed about food served in the facility to know how to complement it with the food they serve at home. If a child has difficulty with any food served at the facility, parents/guardians can address this issue with appropriate staff members. Some regulatory agencies require menus as a part of the licensing and auditing process (2).

COMMENTS: Caregivers/teachers should be aware that new foods may need to be offered between eight to fifteen times before a food may be accepted (3,5). Posting menus in a prominent area and distributing them to parents/guardians helps to inform them about proper nutrition. Sample menus and menu planning templates are available from most state health departments, the state extension service, and the Child and Adult Care Food Program (CACFP).

Good communication between the caregiver/teacher and the parents/guardians is essential for successful feeding, in general, including when introducing age-appropriate solid foods (complementary foods). The decision to feed specific foods should be made in consultation with the parents/guardians. It is recommended that the caregiver/teacher be given written instructions on the introduction and feeding of foods from the parents/guardians and the infant's primary care provider. Caregivers/teachers should use or develop a take-home sheet for parents/guardians on which the caregiver/teacher records the food consumed each day or, for breastfed infants, the number of breastfeedings, and other important notes on the infant. Caregivers/teachers should continue to consult with each infant's parents/guardians concerning foods they have introduced and are feeding. In this way, the caregiver/teacher can follow a schedule of introducing new foods one at a time and more easily identify possible food allergies or intolerances. Caregivers/teachers should let parents/guardians know what and how much their infant eats each day. Consistency between home and the early care and education setting is essential during the period of rapid change when infants are learning to eat age-appropriate solid foods (1,4,6).

RELATED STANDARDS

General Plan for Feeding Infants
Introduction of Age-Appropriate Solid Foods to Infants
Experience with Familiar and New Foods

REFERENCES:

1. Benjamin, S. E., ed. 2007. *Making food healthy and safe for children: How to meet the national health and safety performance standards – Guidelines for out-of-home child care programs*. 2nd ed. Chapel Hill, NC: National Training Institute for Child Care Health Consultants. http://nti.unc.edu/course_files/curriculum/nutrition/making_food_healthy_and_safe.pdf.
2. Benjamin, S. E., K. A. Copeland, A. Cradock, E. Walker, M. M. Slining, B. Neelon, M. W. Gillman. 2009. Menus in child care: A comparison of state regulations to national standards. *J Am Diet Assoc* 109:109-15.
3. Sullivan, S. A., L. L. Birch. 1990. Pass the sugar, pass the salt: Experience dictates preference. *Devel Psych* 26:546-51.
4. U.S. Department of Agriculture, Food and Nutrition Service. 2002. *Feeding infants: A guide for use in the child nutrition programs*. Rev ed. Alexandria, VA: USDA, FNS. http://www.fns.usda.gov/tn/resources/feeding_infants.pdf.
5. Pipes, P. L., C. M. Trahms, eds. 1997. *Nutrition in infancy and childhood*. 6th ed. New York: McGraw-Hill.
6. Grummer-Strawn, L. M., K. S. Scanlon, S. B. Fein. 2008. Infant feeding and feeding transitions during the first year of life. *Pediatrics* 122:S36-42.

Care for Children with Food Allergies

STANDARD: When children with food allergies attend the early care and education facility, the following should occur:

a) Each child with a food allergy should have a care plan prepared for the facility by the child's primary care provider, to include:
   1) Written instructions regarding the food(s) to which the child is allergic and steps that need to be taken to avoid that food;
   2) A detailed treatment plan to be implemented in the event of an allergic reaction, including the names, doses, and methods of administration of any medications that the child should receive in the event of a reaction. The plan should include specific symptoms that would indicate the need to administer one or more medications;

b) Based on the child's care plan, the child's caregivers/teachers should receive training, demonstrate competence in, and implement measures for:
   1) Preventing exposure to the specific food(s) to which the child is allergic;
   2) Recognizing the symptoms of an allergic reaction;
   3) Treating allergic reactions;

c) Parents/guardians and staff should arrange for the facility to have necessary medications, proper storage of such medications, and the equipment and training to manage the child's food allergy while the child is at the early care and education facility;

d) Caregivers/teachers should promptly and properly administer prescribed medications in the event of an allergic reaction according to the instructions in the care plan;

e) The facility should notify the parents/guardians immediately of any suspected allergic reactions, the ingestion of the problem food, or contact with the problem food, even if a reaction did not occur;

f) The facility should recommend to the family that the child's primary care provider be notified if the child has required treatment by the facility for a food allergic reaction;

g) The facility should contact the emergency medical services system immediately whenever epinephrine has been administered;

h) Parents/guardians of all children in the child's class should be advised to avoid any known allergens in class treats or special foods brought into the early care and education setting;

i) Individual child's food allergies should be posted prominently in the classroom where staff can view and/or wherever food is served;

j) The written child care plan, a mobile phone, and the proper medications for appropriate treatment if the child develops an acute allergic reaction should be routinely carried on field trips or transport out of the early care and education setting.

RATIONALE: Food allergy is common, occurring in between 2% and 8% of infants and children (1). Food allergic reactions can range from mild skin or gastrointestinal symptoms to severe, life-threatening reactions with respiratory and/or cardiovascular compromise. Hospitalizations from food allergy are being reported in increasing numbers (5). A major factor in death from anaphylaxis has been a delay in the administration of life-saving emergency medication, particularly epinephrine (6). Intensive efforts to avoid exposure to the offending food(s) are therefore warranted. The maintenance of detailed care plans and the ability to implement such plans for the treatment of reactions are essential for all food-allergic children (2-4).

COMMENTS: Successful food avoidance requires a cooperative effort that must include the parents/guardians, the child, the child's primary care provider, and the early care and education staff. The parents/guardians, with the help of the child's primary care provider, must provide detailed information on the specific foods to be avoided. In some cases, especially for children with multiple food allergies, the parents/guardians may need to take responsibility for providing all of the child's food. In other cases, the early care and education staff may be able to provide safe foods as long as they have been fully educated about effective food avoidance.

Effective food avoidance has several facets. Foods can be listed on an ingredient list under a variety of names, such as milk being listed as casein, caseinate, whey, and/or lactoglobulin. Food sharing between children must be prevented by careful supervision and repeated instruction to the child about this issue. Exposure may also occur through contact between children or by contact with contaminated surfaces, such as a table on which the food allergen remains after eating. Some children may have an allergic reaction just from being in proximity to the offending food, without actually ingesting it. Such contact should be minimized by washing children's hands and faces and all surfaces that were in contact with food. In addition, reactions may occur when a food is used as part of an art or craft project, such as the use of peanut butter to make a bird feeder or wheat to make play dough.

Some children with a food allergy will have mild reactions and will only need to avoid the problem food(s). Others will need to have an antihistamine or epinephrine available to be used in the event of a reaction. For all children with a history of anaphylaxis (severe allergic reaction), or for those with peanut and/or tree nut allergy (whether or not they have had anaphylaxis), epinephrine should be readily available. This will usually be provided as a pre-measured dose in an auto-injector, such as the EpiPen or EpiPen Junior. Specific indications for administration of epinephrine should be provided in the detailed care plan. Within the context of state laws, appropriate personnel should be prepared to administer epinephrine when needed. In virtually all cases, Emergency Medical Services (EMS) should be called immediately and children should be transported to the emergency room by ambulance after the administration of epinephrine. A single dose of epinephrine wears off in fifteen to twenty minutes and many experts will recommend that a second dose be available for administration.

For more information on food allergies, contact the Food Allergy & Anaphylaxis Network or visit their Website at http://www.foodallergy.org/

Some early care and education/school settings require that all foods brought into the classroom are store-bought in their original packaging so that a list of ingredients is included, in order to prevent exposure to allergens.

RELATED STANDARDS:

Assessment and Planning of Nutrition for Individual Children
Feeding Plans and Dietary Modifications

REFERENCES:

1. Burks, A. W., J. S. Stanley. 1998. Food allergy. *Curr Opin Pediatrics* 10:588-93.

2. U.S. Department of Health and Human Services, Administration for Children and Families, Office of Head Start. 2009. *Head Start program performance standards*. Rev. ed. Washington, DC: U.S. Government Printing Office. http://eclkc.ohs.acf.hhs.gov/hslc/Program%20Design%20and%20Management/Head%20Start%20Requirements/Head%20Start%20Requirements/45%20CFR%20Chapter%20XIII/45%20CFR%20Chap%20XIII_ENG.pdf.

3. Kleinman, R. E., ed. 2009. *Pediatric nutrition handbook*. 6th ed. Elk Grove Village, IL: American Academy of Pediatrics.

4. Samour, P. Q., K. King. 2005. *Handbook of pediatric nutrition*. 3rd ed. Lake Dallas, TX: Helm.

5. Branum, A. M., S. L. Lukacs. 2008. *Food allergy among U.S. children: Trends in prevalence and hospitalizations*. NCHS data brief, no. 10. Hyattsville, MD: National Center for Health Statistics.

6. Muraro, A., et at. 2010. The management of the allergic child at school: EAACI/GA2LEN Task Force on the allergic child at school. *Allergy* 65:681-89.

Ingestion of Substances that Do Not Provide Nutrition

STANDARD: All children should be monitored to prevent them from eating substances that do not provide nutrition (often referred to as Pica). The parents/guardians of children who repeatedly place non-nutritive substances in their mouths should be notified and informed of the importance of their child visiting their primary care provider.

RATIONALE: Children who ingest paint chips or contaminated soil can develop lead toxicity which can lead to developmental delays and neurodevelopmental disability. Children who regularly ingest non-nutritive substances can develop iron deficiency anemia. Eating soil or drinking contaminated water could result in an infection with a parasite.

In collaboration with the child's parent/guardian, an assessment of the child's eating behavior and dietary intake should occur along with any other health issues to begin an intervention strategy. Dietary intake plays an important role because certain nutrients such as a diet high in fat or lecithin increase the absorption of lead which can result in toxicity (1).

Currently there is consensus that repeated ingestion of some non-food items results in an increased lead burden of the body (1,2). Early detection and intervention in non-food ingestion can prevent nutritional deficiencies and growth/developmental disabilities.

The occasional ingestion of non-nutritive substances can be a part of everyday living and is not necessarily a concern. For example, ingestion of non-nutritive substances can occur from mouthing, placing dirty hands in the mouth, or eating dropped food. Pica involves the recurrent ingestion of substances that do not provide nutrition. Pica is most prevalent among children between the ages of one and three years (1). Among children with intellectual developmental disability and concurrent mental illness, the incidence exceeds 50% (1).

COMMENTS: Lead-based paint (old housing as well as lead water pipes), neighborhoods with heavy traffic (leaded fuel), and the storage of acidic foods in open cans or ceramic containers with a lead glaze are sources of lead and should be addressed concurrently with a nutritionally adequate diet as prevention strategies. Community water supply may be a source of lead and should be analyzed for its lead content and other metals. Once a child is identified with lead toxicity, it is important to control the child's exposure to the source of lead and promote a healthy and balanced diet. This health problem can be addressed through collaboration among the child's parents/guardians, primary care provider, local childhood lead poisoning prevention program, and the comprehensive child care team of health, education and nutrition staff.

REFERENCES

1. Ekvall, S. W., V. K. Ekvall, eds. 2005. *Pediatric nutrition in chronic disease and developmental disorders: Prevention, assessment, and treatment*. 2nd ed. New York: Oxford University Press.
2. Mitchell, M. K. 2002. *Nutrition across the life span*. 2nd ed. Philadelphia: W. R. Saunders Co.

Vegetarian/Vegan Diets

STANDARD: Infants and children, including school-age children from families practicing any level of vegetarian diet, can be accommodated in an early care and education environment when there is:

a) Written documentation from parents/guardians on the detailed and accurate dietary history about food choices - foods eaten, levels of limitations/restrictions to foods, and frequency of foods offered ;
b) An up-to-date health record of the child available to the caregivers/teachers, including information about linear growth and rate of weight gain, or consistent poor appetite (these indicators can be warning signs of growth deficiencies);
c) Collaboration among early care and education staff, especially the sharing of updated information on the child's health with the parents/guardians by the Child Care Health Consultant and the Nutritionist/Registered Dietitian;
d) Sound health and nutrition information that is culturally relevant to the family to ensure that the child receives adequate calories and essential nutrients which promote adequate growth and development of the child.

RATIONALE: Infants and young children are at highest risk for nutritional deficiencies for energy levels and essential nutrients including protein, calcium, iron, zinc, vitamins B6, B12, and vitamin D (1-3). The younger the child the more critical it is to know about family food choices, limitations and restrictions because the child is dependent on family food (2). Also due to the rapid growth in the early years, it is imperative that a child's diet should consist of a variety of nourishing food to support growth during this critical period. All vegetarian/vegan children should receive multivitamins, especially vitamin D (400 IU of vitamin D are recommended for infants six months to adulthood unless there is certainty of having the daily allowance met by foods); infants under six months who are exclusively or partially breastfed and who receive less than sixteen ounces of formula per day should receive 400 IU of vitamin D (4).

COMMENTS: For older children who have more choice about what they chose to eat and drink, effort should be made to provide accurate nutrition information so they make the wisest food choices for themselves. Both the early care and education program/school and the caregiver/teacher have an opportunity to inform, teach, and promote sound eating practices along with the consequences when poor food choices are made (1). Sensitivity to cultural factors including beliefs and practices of a child's family should be maintained.

Changing lifestyles, convictions and beliefs about food and religion, what is eaten and what foods are restricted or never consumed, have some families with infants and children practicing several levels of vegetarian diets. Some parents/guardians indicate they are vegetarians, semi-vegetarian, or strict vegetarians because they don't or seldom eat meat. Others label themselves lacto-ovo vegetarians, eating or drinking foods such as eggs and dairy products. Still others describe themselves as vegans who restrict themselves strictly to ingesting only plant-based foods, avoiding all and any animal products.

RELATED STANDARDS:

Assessment and Planning of Nutrition for Individual Children
Routine Health Supervision and Growth Monitoring
Use of Soy-based Formula and Soy Milk

REFERENCES:

1. *Kleinman, R. E., ed. 2009. Pediatric nutrition handbook*. 6th ed. Elk Grove Village, IL: American Academy of Pediatrics.
2. Pipes, P. L., C. M. Trahms, eds. 1997. *Nutrition in infancy and childhood*. 6th ed. New York: McGraw-Hill.
3. Mitchell, M. K. 2002. *Nutrition across the life span*. 2nd ed. Philadelphia: W. R. Saunders Co.
4. Wagner, C. L., F. R. Greer. 2008. Prevention of rickets and vitamin D deficiency in infants, children, and adolescents. *Pediatrics* 122:1142–52

Requirements for Infants

General Plan for Feeding Infants

STANDARD: At a minimum, meals and snacks the facility provides for infants should contain the food in the meal and snack patterns of the Child and Adult Care Food Program (CACFP). Food should be appropriate for the infant's individual nutrition requirements and developmental stages as determined by written instructions obtained from the child's parent or primary care provider.

The facility should encourage, provide arrangements for, and support breastfeeding. The facility staff, with appropriate training, should be the mother's cheerleader and enthusiastic supporter for the mother's plan to provide her milk. Facilities should have a designated place set aside for breastfeeding mothers who want to come during work to breastfeed as well as a private area with an outlet (not a bathroom) for mothers to pump their breast milk (2-8). A place that mothers feel they are welcome to breastfeed, pump, or bottle feed can create a positive environment when offered in a supportive way.

Infants may need a variety of special formulas such as soy-based formula or elemental formulas which are easier to digest and less allergenic. Elemental or special non-allergic formulas should be specified in the infant's care plan.

Age-appropriate solid foods (complementary foods) may be introduced no sooner than when the child has reached the age of four months, but preferably six months and as indicated by the individual child's nutritional and developmental needs. For breastfed infants, gradual introduction of iron-fortified foods may occur no sooner than around four months, but preferably six months to complement the human milk.

RATIONALE: Human milk, as an exclusive food, is best suited to meet the entire nutritional needs of an infant from birth until six months of age, with the exception of recommended vitamin D supplementation. In addition to nutrition, breastfeeding supports optimal health and development. Human milk is also the best source of milk for infants for at least the first twelve months of age and, thereafter, for as long as mutually desired by mother and child. Breastfeeding protects infants from many acute and chronic diseases and has advantages for the mother, as well (4).

Research overwhelmingly shows that exclusive breastfeeding for six months, and continued breastfeeding for at least a year or longer, dramatically improves health outcomes for children and their mothers. *Healthy People 2010* Objective 16 includes increasing the proportion of mothers who breastfeed their infants, and increasing the duration of breastfeeding and of exclusively breastfeeding (1).

Importance of breastfeeding to the infant includes reduction of some of the risks that are greater for infants in group care. Many advantages of breastfeeding are documented by research, including reduction in the incidence of diarrhea, respiratory disease, otitis media, bacteremia, bacterial meningitis, botulism, urinary tract infections, necrotizing enterocolitis, SIDS, insulin-dependent diabetes, lymphoma, allergic disease, ulcerative colitis, ear infections, and other chronic digestive diseases (4,13,15). Evidence suggests that breastfeeding is associated with enhanced cognitive development (6,10). Additionally, some evidence suggests that breastfeeding reduces the risk of childhood obesity (9,11). Breastfeeding also lowers the mother's risk of diabetes, breast cancer, and heart disease (17).

Except in the presence of rare genetic diseases, the clear advantage of human milk over any formula should lead to vigorous efforts by caregivers/teachers to promote and sustain breastfeeding for mothers who are willing to nurse their infants whenever they can, and to pump and supply their milk to the early care and education facility when direct feeding from the breast is not possible. Even if infants receive formula during the child care day, some breastfeeding or expressed human milk from their mothers is beneficial (8).

Iron-fortified infant formula is an acceptable alternative to human milk as a food for infant feeding even though it lacks any anti-infective or immunological components. An adequately nourished infant is more likely to achieve normal physical and mental development, which will have long-term positive consequences on health (12,13).

COMMENTS: Some ways to help a mother to breastfeed successfully in the early care and education facility (3):

a) If she wishes to breastfeed her infant or child when she comes to the facility, offer or provide her a:
   1) Quiet, comfortable, and private place to breastfeed (this helps her milk to letdown);
   2) Place to wash her hands;
   3) Pillow to support her infant on her lap while nursing if requested;
   4) Nursing stool or stepstool if requested for her feet

so she doesn't have to strain her back while nursing; and

5) Glass of water or other liquid to help her stay hydrated;

b) Encourage her to get the infant used to being fed her expressed human milk by another person before the infant starts in early care and education, while continuing to breastfeed directly herself;

c) Discuss with her the infant's usual feeding pattern and whether she wants the caregiver/teacher to feed the infant by cue or on a schedule, also ask her if she wishes to time the infant's last feeding so that the infant is hungry and ready to breastfeed when she arrives, also, ask her to leave her availability schedule with the early care and education program and ask her to call if she is planning to miss a feeding or is going to be late;

d) Encourage her to provide a back-up supply of frozen or refrigerated expressed human milk with the infant's full name on the bottle or other clean storage container in case the infant needs to eat more often than usual or the mother's visit is delayed;

e) Share with her information about other places in the community that can answer her questions and concerns about breastfeeding for example, local lactation consultants (14,16);

f) Ensure that all staff receive training in breastfeeding support and promotion;

g) Ensure that all staff are trained in the proper handling and feeding of each milk product, including human milk or infant formula;

h) Provide culturally appropriate breastfeeding materials including community resources for parents/guardians that include appropriate language and pictures of multicultural families to assist families to identify with them.

RELATED STANDARDS:

Written Menus and Introduction of New Foods
Preparing, Feeding, and Storing Human Milk
Preparing, Feeding, and Storing Infant Formula
Introduction of Age-Appropriate Solid Foods to Infants
Feeding Age-Appropriate Solid Foods to Infants
Appendix – Our Child Care Center Supports Breastfeeding

REFERENCES:

1. U.S. Department of Health and Human Services. 2000. *Healthy people 2010: Understanding and improving health*. 2nd ed. Washington, DC: U.S. Government Printing Office. http://www.healthypeople.gov/Document/pdf/uih/2010uih.pdf.
2. Dietitians of Canada, American Dietetic Association. 2000. *Manual of clinical dietetics*. 6th ed. Chicago: ADA.
3. U.S. Department of Agriculture, Food and Nutrition Service. 1993. *Breastfed babies welcome here!* Alexandria, VA: USDA, FNS.
4. American Academy of Pediatrics, Section on Breastfeeding. 2005. Policy statement: Breastfeeding and the use of human milk. *Pediatrics* 115:496-506.
5. Uauy, R., I. DeAndroca. 1995. Human milk and breast feeding for optimal brain development. *J Nutr* 125:2278-80.
6. Wang, Y. S., S. Y. Wu. 1996. The effect of exclusive breast feeding on development and incidence of infection in infants. *J Hum Lactation* 12:2730.
7. Quasdt, S. 1998. Ecology of breast feeding in the US: An applied perspective. *Am J Hum Biol* 10:221-28.
8. Hammosh, M. 1996. Breast feeding and the working mother. *Pediatrics* 97:492-8.
9. Kramer M. S. , L. Matush L, I. Vanilovich I, et al. 2007. Effects of prolonged and exclusive breastfeeding on child height, weight, adiposity, and blood pressure at age 6.5 y: Evidence from a large randomized trial. *Am J Clin Nutr* 86:1717–21.
10. Lawrence, R. A., R. Lawrence. 2005. *Breast feeding: A guide for the medical profession*. 6th ed. St. Louis: Mosby.
11. Birch, L., W. Dietz, eds. 2008. *Eating behaviors of the young child: Prenatal and postnatal influences on healthy eating*. Elk Grove Village, IL: American Academy of Pediatrics.
12. Dietz, W. H., L. Stern, eds. 1998. *American Academy of Pediatrics guide to your child's nutrition*. New York: Villard.
13. Kleinman, R. E., ed. 2009. *Pediatric nutrition handbook*. 6th ed. Elk Grove Village, IL: American Academy of Pediatrics.
14. U.S. Department of Agriculture, Food and Nutrition Service. 2002. *Feeding infants: A guide for use in the child nutrition programs*. Rev ed. Alexandria, VA: USDA, FNS. http://www.fns.usda.gov/tn/resources/feeding_infants.pdf.
15. Ip, S., M. Chung, G. Raman, P. Chew, N. Magula, D. DeVine, T. Trikalinos, J. Lau. 2007. *Breastfeeding and maternal and infant health outcomes in developed countries*. Rockville, MD: Agency for Healthcare Research and Quality.
16. U.S. Department of Agriculture, Food and Nutrition Service. *Benefits and services: Breastfeeding promotion and support in WIC*. http://www.fns.usda.gov/wic/breastfeeding/breastfeedingmainpage.HTM.
17. Stuebe, A. M., E. B. Schwarz. 2009. The risks and benefits of infant feeding practices for women and their children. *J Perinatology* (July 16).

Feeding Infants on Cue by a Consistent Caregiver/Teacher

STANDARD: Caregivers/teachers should feed infants on the infant's cue unless the parent/guardian and the child's primary care provider give written instructions otherwise (6). Whenever possible, the same caregiver/teacher should feed a specific infant for most of that infant's feedings. Cues such as opening the mouth, making suckling sounds, and moving the hands at random all send information from an infant to a caregiver/teacher that the infant is ready to feed. Caregivers/teachers should not feed infants beyond satiety, just as hunger cues are important in initiating feedings, observing satiety cues can limit overfeeding.

RATIONALE: Cue feeding meets the infant's nutritional and emotional needs and provides an immediate response to the infant, which helps ensure trust and feelings of security. Cues such as turning away from the nipple, increased attention to surroundings, keeping mouth closed, and saying no are all indications of satiation (1,2,6). When the same caregiver/teacher regularly works with a particular child, that caregiver/teacher is more likely to understand that child's cues and to respond appropriately. Feeding infants on cue rather than on a schedule may help prevent childhood obesity (3,6). Early relationships between an infant and caregivers/teachers involving feeding set the stage for an infant to develop eating patterns for life (1,4).

COMMENTS: Caregivers/teachers should be gentle, patient, sensitive, and reassuring by responding appropriately to the infant's feeding cues (1). Waiting for an infant to cry to indicate hunger is not necessary or desirable. Crying may indicate that feeding cues have been missed and adequate attention has not been paid to the infant (5). Nevertheless, feeding children who are alert and interested in interpersonal interaction, but who are not showing signs of hunger, is not appropriate. Cues for hunger or interaction-seeking may vary widely in different infants. A pacifier should not be offered to a hungry infant, they need food first.

A series of trainings on infant cues can be found at NCAST-AVENUW, University of Washington at http://www.ncast.org/index.cfm?fuseaction=category.display&category_id=16.

RELATED STANDARRDS:
General Plan for Feeding Infants
Techniques for Bottle Feeding

REFERENCES:
1. Branscomb, K. R., C. B. Goble. 2008. Infants and toddlers in group care: Feeding practices that foster emotional health. *Young Children* 63:28-33.
2. Trahms, C. M., P. L. Pipes, eds. 1997. *Nutrition and infancy in childhood.* 6th ed. New York: McGraw-Hill.
3. Taveras, E. M., S. L. Rifas-Shiman, K. S. Scanlon, L. M. Grummer-Strawn, B. Sherry, M. W. Gillman. 2006. To what extent is the protective effect of breastfeeding on future overweight explained by decreased maternal feeding restriction? *Pediatrics* 118:2341-48.
4. Hodges, E. A., S. O. Hughes, J. Hopkinson, J. O. Fisher. 2008. Maternal decisions about the initiation and termination of infant feeding. *Appetite* 50:333-39.
5. Hagan, J. F., J. S. Shaw, P. M. Duncan, eds. 2008. *Bright futures: Guidelines for health supervision of infants, children, and adolescents.* 3rd ed. Elk Grove Village, IL: American Academy of Pediatrics.
6. Satter, E. 2000. *Child of mine: Feeding with love and good sense.* 3rd ed. Boulder, CO: Bull Publishing.

Preparing, Feeding, and Storing Human Milk

STANDARD: Expressed human milk should be placed in a clean and sanitary bottle with a nipple that fits tightly or into an equivalent clean and sanitary sealed container to prevent spilling during transport to home or to the facility. Only cleaned and sanitized bottles, or their equivalent, and nipples should be used in feeding. The bottle or container should be properly labeled with the infant's full name and the date and time the milk was expressed. The bottle or container should immediately be stored in the refrigerator on arrival.

The mother's own expressed milk should only be used for her own infant. Likewise, infant formula should not be used for a breastfed infant without the mother's written permission.

Bottles made of plastics containing BPA or phthalates should be avoided (labeled with #3, #6, or #7). Glass bottles or plastic bottles labeled BPA Free or with a #1, #2, #4, or #5 are acceptable.

Non-frozen human milk should be transported and stored in the containers to be used to feed the infant, identified with a label which won't come off in water or handling, bearing the date of collection and child's full name. The filled, labeled containers of human milk should be kept refrigerated. Human milk containers with significant amount of contents remaining (greater than one ounce) may be returned to the mother at the end of the day as long as the child has not fed directly from the bottle.

Frozen human milk may be transported and stored in single use plastic bags and placed in a freezer (not a compartment within a refrigerator but either a freezer with a separate door or a standalone freezer). Human milk should be defrosted in the refrigerator if frozen, and then heated briefly in bottle warmers or under warm running water so that the temperature does not exceed 98.6°F. If there is insufficient time to defrost the milk in the refrigerator before warming it, then it may be defrosted in a container of running cool tap water, very gently swirling the bottle periodically to evenly distribute the temperature in the milk. Some infants will not take their mother's milk unless it is warmed to body temperature, around 98.6°F. The caregiver/teacher should check for the infant's full name and the date on the bottle so that the oldest milk is used first. After warming, bottles should be mixed gently (not shaken) and the temperature of the milk tested before feeding.

Expressed human milk that presents a threat to an infant, such as human milk that is in an unsanitary bottle, is curdled, smells rotten, and/or has not been stored following the storage guidelines of the Academy of Breastfeeding Medicine as shown later in this standard, should be returned to the mother.

Some children around six months to a year of age may be developmentally ready to feed themselves and may want to drink from a cup. The transition from bottle to cup can come at a time when a child's fine motor skills allow use of a cup. The caregiver/teacher should use a clean small cup without cracks or chips and should help the child to lift and tilt the cup to avoid spillage and leftover fluid. The caregiver/teacher and mother should work together on cup feeding of human milk to ensure the child is receiving adequate nourishment and to avoid having a large amount of human milk remaining at the end of feeding. Two to three ounces of human milk can be placed in a clean cup and additional milk can be offered as needed. Small amounts of human milk (about an ounce) can be discarded.

Human milk can be stored using the following guidelines from the Academy of Breastfeeding Medicine:

Guidelines for Storage of Human Milk

Location	Temperature	Duration	Comments
Countertop, table	Room temperature (up to 77°F or 25°C)	6-8 hours	Containers should be covered and kept as cool as possible; covering the container with a cool towel may keep milk cooler.
Insulated cooler bag	5°F– 39°F or -15°C–4°C	24 hours	Keep ice packs in contact with milk containers at all times, limit opening cooler bag.
Refrigerator	39°F or 4°C	5 days	Store milk in the back of the main body of the refrigerator.
Freezer			Store milk toward the back of the freezer, where temperature is most constant. Milk stored for longer durations in the ranges listed is safe, but some of the lipids in the milk undergo degradation resulting in lower quality.
Freezer compartment of a refrigerator	5°F or -15°C	2 weeks	
Freezer compartment of refrigerator with separate doors	0°F or -18°C	3-6 months	
Chest or upright deep freezer	-4°F or -20°C	6-12 months	

Source: Academy of Breastfeeding Medicine. 2010. Clinical protocol #8: Human milk storage information for home use for healthy full term infants. Rev. ed. Princeton Junction, NJ: ABM. http://www.bfmed.org/Resources/Download.aspx?filename=Protocol 8 - English.pdf.
From the Centers for Disease Control and Prevention Website: Proper handling and storage of human milk – Storage duration of fresh human milk for use with healthy full term infants. http://www.cdc.gov/breastfeeding/recommendations/handling_breastmilk.htm.

RATIONALE: Labels for containers of human milk should be resistant to loss of the name and date/time when washing and handling. This is especially important when the frozen bottle is thawed in running tap water. There may be several bottles from different mothers being thawed and warmed at the same time in the same place.

By following this standard, the staff is able, when necessary, to prepare human milk and feed an infant safely, thereby reducing the risk of inaccuracy or feeding the infant unsanitary or incorrect human milk (2,5).

Written guidance for both staff and parents/guardians should be available to determine when milk provided by parents/guardians will not be served. Human milk cannot be served if it does not meet the requirements for sanitary and safe milk.

Excessive shaking of human milk may damage some of the cellular components that are valuable to the infant.

It is difficult to maintain 0°F consistently in a freezer compartment of a refrigerator or freezer, so caregivers/teachers should carefully monitor, with daily log sheets, temperature of freezers used to store human milk using an appropriate working thermometer. Human milk contains components that are damaged by excessive heating during or after thawing from the frozen state (1). Currently, there is nothing in the research literature that states that feedings must be warmed at all prior to feeding. Frozen milk should never be thawed in a microwave oven as 1) uneven hot spots in the milk may cause burns in the infant and 2) excessive heat may destroy beneficial components of the milk.

By following safe preparation and storage techniques, nursing mothers and caregivers/teachers of breastfed infants and children can maintain the high quality of expressed human milk and the health of the infant (3,4,6).

COMMENTS: Although human milk is a body fluid, it is not necessary to wear gloves when feeding or handling human milk. Unless there is visible blood in the milk, the risk of exposure to infectious organisms either during feeding or from milk that the infant regurgitates is not significant.

Returning unused human milk to the mother informs her of the quantity taken while in the early care and education program.

RELATED STANDARDS:

General Plan for Feeding Infants
Feeding Cow's Milk
Feeding Human Milk to Another Mother's Child
Techniques for Bottle Feeding
Warming Bottles and Infant Foods

REFERENCES:

1. American Academy of Pediatrics, Section on Breastfeeding. 2005. Policy statement: Breastfeeding and the use of human milk. *Pediatrics* 115:496-506.
2. Clark, A., J. Anderson, E. Adams, S. Baker. 2008. Assessing the knowledge, attitudes, behaviors and training needs related to infant feeding, specifically breastfeeding, of child care providers. *Matern Child Health J* 12:128-35.
3. Kleinman, R. E., ed. 2009. *Pediatric nutrition handbook*. 6th ed. Elk Grove Village, IL: American Academy of Pediatrics.
4. Samour, P. Q., K. King. 2005. *Handbook of pediatric nutrition*. 3rd ed. Lake Dallas, TX: Helm.
5. Lawrence, R. A., R. Lawrence. 2005. *Breast feeding: A guide for the medical profession*. 6th ed. St. Louis: Mosby.
6. Endres, J. B., R. E. Rockwell. 2003. *Food, nutrition, and the young child*. 4th ed. New York: Macmillan.

Feeding Human Milk to Another Mother's Child

STANDARD: If a child has been mistakenly fed another child's bottle of expressed human milk, the possible exposure to hepatitis B, hepatitis C, or HIV should be treated as if an exposure to other body fluids had occurred. For possible exposure to hepatitis B, hepatitis C, or HIV, the caregiver/teacher should:

a) Inform the mother who expressed the human milk about the mistake and when the bottle switch occurred, and ask:
   1) When the human milk was expressed and how it was handled prior to being delivered to the caregiver/teacher or facility;
   2) Whether she has ever had a hepatitis B, hepatitis C, or HIV blood test and, if so, the date of the test and would she be willing to share the results with the parents/guardians of the child who was fed the incorrect milk;
   3) If she does not know whether she has ever been tested for hepatitis B, hepatitis C, or HIV, would she be willing to contact her primary care provider and find out if she has been tested;
   4) If she has never been tested for hepatitis B, hepatitis C, or HIV, would she be willing to be tested and share the results with the parents/guardians of the other child;

b) Discuss the mistake of giving the wrong milk with the parents/guardians of the child who was fed the wrong bottle:
   1) Inform them that their child was given another child's bottle of expressed human milk and the date it was given;
   2) Inform them that the risk of transmission of hepatitis B, hepatitis C, or HIV and other infectious diseases is low;
   3) Encourage the parents/guardians to notify the child's primary care provider of the exposure;
   4) Provide the family with information including the time at which the milk was expressed and how the milk was handled prior to its being delivered to the caregiver/teacher so that the parents/guardians may inform the child's primary care provider;

5) Inform the parents/guardians that, depending upon the results from the mother whose milk was given mistakenly (1), their child may soon need to undergo a baseline blood test for hepatitis B (also see below), hepatitis C, or HIV;

c) Assess why the wrong milk was given and develop a prevention plan to be shared with the parents/guardians as well as the staff in the facility.

If the human milk given mistakenly to a child is from a woman who does not know her hepatitis B status, the caregiver/teacher should determine if the child has received the complete hepatitis B vaccine series. If the child has not been vaccinated or is incompletely vaccinated, then the parent of the child who received the milk should seek vaccination of the child. The child should complete the recommended childhood hepatitis B vaccine series as soon as possible. If human milk from a hepatitis B-positive woman is given mistakenly to a an unimmunized child, the child may receive HBIG (Hepatitis B Immune Globulin) as soon as possible within seven days, but it is not necessary because of the low risk of transmission (3). The hepatitis B vaccine series should be initiated and completed as soon as possible.

RATIONALE: The risk of hepatitis B, hepatitis C, or HIV transmission from expressed human milk consumed by another child is believed to be low because:

a) In the United States, women who are HIV-positive and aware of that fact, are advised NOT to breastfeed their infants and therefore the potential for exposure to milk from an HIV-positive woman is low;

b) In the United States, women with high hepatitis C antiviral loads or who have cracked or bleeding nipples might transmit the infection through breastfeeding. Therefore, they are advised to refrain from breastfeeding (3,4);

c) Chemicals present in human milk act, together with time and cold temperatures, to destroy the HIV present in expressed human milk;

d) Transmission of HIV from a single human milk exposure has never been documented (1).

Because parents/guardians may express concern about the likelihood of transmitting these diseases through human milk, this issue is addressed in detail to assure there is a very small risk of such transmission occurring.

Among known HIV-positive women in Africa (where HIV-positive women are still advised to breastfeed only if they are located in areas where the water supply is unreliable), a study found that the transmission rate among infants who were fed infected human milk exclusively for several months was found to be 4%; thirteen infants out of 324 (2).

RELATED STANDARDS:

Preparing, Feeding, and Storing Human Milk

REFERENCES:

1. Centers for Disease Control and Prevention. *What to do if an infant or child is mistakenly fed another woman's expressed breast milk.* http://www.cdc.gov/breastfeeding/recommendations/other_mothers_milk.htm#.

2. Becquet, R., D. K. Ekouevi, H. Menan, C. Amani-Bosse, L. Bequet, I. Viho, F. Dabis, M. Timite-Konan, V. Leroy. 2008. Early mixed feeding and breastfeeding beyond 6 months increase the risk of postnatal HIV transmission. *Prev Med* 47:27-33.

3. Pickering, L. K., C. J. Baker, D. W. Kimberlin, S. J. Long. 2009. *Red Book 2009: Report of the Committee on Infectious Diseases.* Elk Grove Village, IL: American Academy of Pediatrics.

4. Philip Spradling, CDC, e-mail message to the NRC, May 12, 2010.

Preparing, Feeding, and Storing Infant Formula

STANDARD: Formula provided by parents/guardians or by the facility should come in a factory-sealed container. The formula should be of the same brand that is served at home and should be of ready-to-feed strength or liquid concentrate to be diluted using water from a source approved by the health department. Powdered infant formula, though it is the least expensive formula, requires special handling in mixing because it cannot be sterilized. The primary source for proper and safe handling and mixing is the manufacturer's instructions that appear on the can of powdered formula. Before opening the can, hands should be washed. The can and plastic lid should be thoroughly rinsed and dried. Caregivers/teachers should read and follow the manufacturer's directions. If instructions are not readily available, caregivers/teachers should obtain information from the World Health Organization's *Safe Preparation, Storage and Handling of Powdered Infant Formula Guidelines* at http://www.who.int/foodsafety/publications/micro/pif2007/en/index.html. The local WIC program can also provide instructions.

Formula mixed with cereal, fruit juice, or any other foods should not be served unless the child's primary care provider provides written documentation that the child has a medical reason for this type of feeding.

Iron-fortified formula should be refrigerated until immediately before feeding. For bottles containing formula, any contents remaining after a feeding should be discarded.

Bottles of formula prepared from powder or concentrate or ready-to-feed formula should be labeled with the child's full name and date of preparation. Prepared formula must be discarded within one hour after serving to an infant. Prepared formula that has not been given to an infant may be stored in the refrigerator for twenty-four hours to prevent bacterial contamination. An open container of ready-to-feed, concentrated formula, or formula prepared from concentrated formula, should be covered, refrigerated, and discarded at forty-eight hours if not used.

Some infants will require specialized formula because of allergy, inability to digest certain formulas, or need for extra calories. The appropriate formula should always be available and should be fed as directed. For those infants getting supplemental calories, the formula may be prepared in a different way from the directions on the container. In those circumstances, either the family should provide the prepared formula or the caregiver/teacher should receive special training, as noted in the infant's care plan, on how to prepare the formula.

RATIONALE: This standard promotes the feeding of infant formula that is familiar to the infant and supports family feeding practice. By following this standard, the staff is able, when necessary, to prepare formula and feed an infant safely, thereby reducing the risk of inaccuracy or feeding the infant unsanitary or incorrect formula. Written guidance for both staff and parents/guardians must be available to determine when formula provided by parents/guardians will not be served. Formula cannot be served if it does not meet the requirements for sanitary and safe formula.

If a child has a special health problem, such as reflux, or inability to take in nutrients because of delayed development of feeding skills, the child's primary care provider should provide a written plan for the staff to follow so that the child is fed appropriately. Some infants are allergic to milk and soy and need to be fed an elemental formula which does not contain allergens. Other infants need supplemental calories because of poor weight gain.

Infants should not be fed a formula different from the one the parents/guardians feed at home, as even minor differences in formula can cause gastrointestinal upsets and other problems (6).

Excessive shaking of formula may cause foaming that increases the likelihood of feeding air to the infant.

Formula should not be used beyond the stated shelf life period (1).

COMMENTS: The intent of this standard is to protect a child's health by ensuring safe and sanitary conditions for transporting and feeding infant formula prepared at home and brought to the facility, and by ensuring that all infants get the proper formula.

The bottles must be sanitary, properly prepared and stored, and must be the same brand in the early care and education program and at home.

Staff preparing formula should thoroughly wash their hands prior to beginning preparation of infant feedings of any type. Water used for mixing infant formula must be from a safe water source as defined by the local or state health department. If the caregiver/teacher is concerned or uncertain about the safety of the tap water, she/he may use bottled water or bring cold tap water to a rolling boil for one minute (no longer), then cool the water to room temperature for no more than thirty minutes before it is used. Warmed water should be tested in advance to make sure it is not too hot for the infant. To test the temperature, the caregiver/teacher should shake a few drops on the inside of her/his wrist. A bottle can be prepared by adding powdered formula and room temperature water from the tap just before feeding. Bottles made in this way from powdered formula can be ready for feeding as no additional refrigeration or warming would be required.

Caregivers/teachers should only use the scoop that comes with the can and not interchange the scoop from one product to another, since the volume of the scoop may vary from manufacturer to manufacturer and product to product. Also, a scoop can be contaminated with a potential allergen from another type of formula. Although many infant formulas are made from powder, the liquid preparations are diluted with water at the factory. Concentrated infant formula, not ready-to feed, must be diluted with water. Sealed, ready-to-feed bottles are easy to use, however they are the most expensive approach to feeding formula.

If concentrated liquid or powdered infant formulas are used, it is very important to prepare them properly, with accurate dilution, according to the directions on the container. Adding too little water to formula puts a burden on an infant's kidneys and digestive system and may lead to dehydration (4). Adding too much water dilutes the formula. Diluted formula may interfere with an infant's growth and health because it provides inadequate calories and nutrients and can cause water intoxication. Water intoxication can occur in breastfed or formula-fed infants or children over one year of age who are fed an excessive amount of water. Water intoxication can be life-threatening to an infant or young child (5).

RELATED STANDARDS:
General Plan for Feeding Infants
Techniques for Bottle Feeding
Warming Bottles and Infant Food

REFERENCES:
1. Kleinman, R. E., ed. 2009. *Pediatric nutrition handbook*. 6th ed. Elk Grove Village, IL: American Academy of Pediatrics.
2. Dietitians of Canada, American Dietetic Association. 2000. *Manual of clinical dietetics*. 6th ed. Chicago: ADA.
3. Pipes, P. L., C. M. Trahms, eds. 1997. *Nutrition in infancy and childhood*. 6th ed. New York: McGraw-Hill.
4. University of Wisconsin-Madison. Food facts for you: Safe preparation of infant formula. http://www.foodsafety.wisc.edu/assets/food-facts_2004/wffjune2004.htm#Infant.
5. U.S. Department of Agriculture, Food and Nutrition Service. 2002. *Feeding infants: A guide for use in the child nutrition programs*. Rev ed. Alexandria, VA: USDA, FNS. http://www.fns.usda.gov/tn/resources/feeding_infants.pdf.
6. American Academy of Pediatrics, Section on Breastfeeding. 2005. Policy statement: Breastfeeding and the use of human milk. *Pediatrics* 115:496-506.

Techniques for Bottle Feeding

STANDARD: Infants should always be held for bottle feeding. Caregivers/teachers should hold infants in the caregiver/teacher's arms or sitting up on the caregiver/teacher's lap. Bottles should never be propped. The facility should not permit infants to have bottles in the crib. The facility should not permit an infant to carry a bottle while standing, walking, or running around.

Bottle feeding techniques should mimic approaches to breastfeeding:

a) Initiate feeding when infant provides cues (rooting, sucking, etc.);
b) Hold the infant during feedings and respond to vocalizations with eye contact and vocalizations;
c) Alternate sides of caregiver's/teacher's lap;
d) Allow breaks during the feeding for burping;
e) Allow infant to stop the feeding.

A caregiver/teacher should not bottle feed more than one infant at a time.

Bottles should be checked to ensure they are given to the appropriate child, have human milk, infant formula, or water in them.

When using a bottle for a breastfed infant, a nipple with a cylindrical teat and a wider base is usually preferable. A shorter or softer nipple may be helpful for infants with a hypersensitive gag reflex, or those who cannot get their lips well back on the wide base of the teat (22).

The use of a bottle or cup to modify or pacify a child's behavior should not be allowed (1,16).

RATIONALE: The manner in which food is given to infants is conducive to the development of sound eating habits for life. Caregivers/teachers should promote proper feeding practices and oral hygiene including proper use of the bottle for all infants and toddlers. Bottle propping can cause choking and aspiration and may contribute to long-term health issues, including ear infections (otitis media), orthodontic problems, speech disorders, and psychological problems (1-6). When infants and children are "cue fed", they are in control of frequency and amount of feedings. This has been found to reduce the risk of childhood obesity.

Any liquid except plain water can cause early childhood caries (7-18). Early childhood caries in primary teeth may hold significant short-term and long-term implications for the child's health (7-18). Frequently sipping any liquid besides plain water between feeds encourages tooth decay.

Children are at an increased risk for injury when they walk around with bottle nipples in their mouths. Bottles should not be allowed in the crib or bed for safety and sanitary reasons and for preventing dental caries. It is difficult for a caregiver/teacher to be aware of and respond to infant feeding cues when feeding more than one infant at a time.

COMMENTS: Caregivers/teachers and parents/guardians need to understand the relationship between bottle feeding and emotional security. Caregivers/teachers should hold infants who are bottle feeding whenever possible, even if the children are old enough to hold their own bottle.

Caregivers/teachers should offer children fluids from a cup as soon as they are developmentally ready. Some children may be able to drink from a cup around six months of age, while for others, it is later (2). Weaning a child to drink from a cup is an individual process, which occurs over a wide range of time. The American Academy of Pediatric Dentistry (AAPD) recommends weaning from a bottle by the child's first birthday (1-3,6-9). Instead of sippy cups, caregivers /teachers should use smaller cups and fill halfway or less to prevent spills as children learn to use a cup (19-21). If sippy cups are used, it should only be for a very short transition period.

Some children around six months to a year of age may be developmentally ready to feed themselves and may want to drink from a cup. The transition from bottle to cup can come at a time when a child's fine motor skills allow use of a cup. The caregiver/teacher should use a clean small cup without cracks or chips and should help the child to lift and tilt the cup to avoid spillage and leftover fluid. The caregiver/teacher and parent/guardian should work together on cup feeding of human milk to ensure the child's receiving adequate nourishment and to avoid having a large amount of human milk remaining at the end of feeding. Two to three ounces of human milk can be placed in a clean cup and additional milk can be offered as needed. Small amounts of human milk (about an ounce) can be discarded.

Infants should be burped after every feeding and preferably during the feeding as well.

RELATED STANDARDS:

Feeding Infants on Cue by a Consistent Caregiver/Teacher
Techniques for Bottle Feeding
Warming Bottles and Infant Foods

REFERENCES:

1. Kleinman, R. E., ed. 2009. *Pediatric nutrition handbook*. 6th ed. Elk Grove Village, IL: American Academy of Pediatrics.
2. Casamassimo, P., K. Holt, eds. 2004. *Bright futures in practice: Oral health–pocket guide*. Washington, DC: National Maternal and Child Oral Health Resource Center. http://www.mchoralhealth.org/PDFs/BFOHPocketGuide.pdf.
3. Dietitians of Canada, American Dietetic Association. 2000. *Manual of clinical dietetics*. 6th ed. Chicago: ADA.
4. Wang, Y. S., S. Y. Wu. 1996. The effect of exclusive breast feeding on development and incidence of infection in infants. *J Hum Lactation* 12:2730.
5. American Academy of Pediatric Dentistry. 1993. Recommendation for preventive pediatric dental care. *Pediatr Dent* 15:158-59.
6. American Academy of Pediatric Dentistry. 1994. Reference manual, 1994-1995. *Pediatr Dent* 16:196.
7. Schafer, T. E., S. M. Adair. 2000. Prevention of dental disease: The role of the pediatrician. *Pediatr Clin North Am* 47:1021-42.
8. Ramos-Gomez, F. J. 2005. Clinical considerations for an infant oral health care program. *Compend Contin Educ Dent* 26:17-23.
9. Ramos-Gomez, F. J., B. Jue, C. Y. Bonta. 2002. Implementing an infant oral care program. *J Calif Dent Assoc* 30:752-61.
10. U.S. Department of Health and Human Services. 2000. *Oral health in America: A report of the surgeon general–Executive summary*. Rockville, MD: U.S. Department of Health and Human Services, National Institute of Dental and Craniofacial Research, National Institutes of Health.
11. Section on Pediatric Dentistry and Oral Health. 2008. Preventive oral health intervention for pediatricians. *Pediatrics* 122:1387-94.
12. New York State Department of Health. 2006. Oral health care during pregnancy and early childhood: Practice guidelines. Albany, NY: New York State Department of Health. http://www.health.state.ny.us/publications/0824.pdf.
13. American Dental Association. 2004. From baby bottle to cup: Choose training cups carefully, use them temporarily. *J Am Dent Assoc* 135:387.
14. American Dental Association. ADA statement on early childhood caries. http://www.ada.org/2057.aspx.
15. The American Academy of Pediatric Dentistry. 2002. Policy on baby bottle tooth decay (BBTD)/early childhood caries (ECC): Reference Manual 2002-2003. http://www.aapd.org/members/referencemanual/pdfs/02-03/Baby%20Bottle%20Tooth%20Decay.pdf.
16. American Academy of Pediatrics. 2007. Brushing up on oral health: Never too early to start. *Healthy Children* (Winter): 14-15. http://www.aap.org/family/healthychildren/07winter/oralhealth.pdf.
17. Tinanoff, N., C. Palmer. 2000. Dietary determinants of dental caries and dietary recommendations for preschool children. *J Public Health Dent* 60:197-206.
18. Pipes, P. L., C. M. Trahms, eds. 1997. *Nutrition in infancy and childhood*. 6th ed. New York: McGraw-Hill.
19. Prolonged use of sippy cups under scrutiny. 2002. *Dentistry Today* 21:44.
20. Behrendt, A., F. Szlegoleit, V. Muler-Lessmann, G. Ipek-Ozdemir, W. F. Wetzel. 2001. Nursing-bottle syndrome caused by prolonged drinking from vessels with bill-shaped extensions. *ASDC J Dent Child* 68:47-54.
21. Satter, E. 2000. *Child of mine: Feeding with love and good sense*. 3rd ed. Boulder, CO: Bull Publishing.
22. Watson Genna, C. 2008. *Supporting sucking skills in breastfeeding infants*. Sudbury, MA: Jones and Bartlett.

Warming Bottles and Infant Foods

STANDARD: Bottles and infant foods can be served cold from the refrigerator and do not have to be warmed. If a caregiver/teacher chooses to warm them, bottles should be warmed under running, warm tap water or by placing them in a container of water that is no warmer than 120°F. Bottles should not be left in a pot of water to warm for more than five minutes. Bottles and infant foods should never be warmed in a microwave oven.

Infant foods should be stirred carefully to distribute the heat evenly. A caregiver/teacher should not hold an infant while removing a bottle or infant food from the container of warm water or while preparing a bottle or stirring infant food that has been warmed in some other way. Only BPA-free plastic, plastic labeled #1,#2,#4 or#5, or glass bottles should be used.

If a slow-cooking device, such as a crock pot, is used for warming infant formula, human milk, or infant food, this slow-cooking device should be out of children's reach, should contain water at a temperature that does not exceed 120°F, and should be emptied, cleaned, sanitized, and refilled with fresh water daily.

RATIONALE: Bottles of human milk or infant formula that

are warmed at room temperature or in warm water for an extended time provide an ideal medium for bacteria to grow. Infants have received burns from hot water dripping from an infant bottle that was removed from a crock pot or by pulling the crock pot down on themselves by a dangling cord. Caution should be exercised to avoid raising the water temperature above a safe level for warming infant formula or infant food. Human milk, formula, or food fed to infants should never be heated in a microwave oven as uneven hot spots in milk and/or food may burn the infant (1,2).

RELATED STANDARDS:
Techniques for Bottle Feeding
Feeding Age-Appropriate Solid Foods to Infants

REFERENCES:
1. Nemethy, M., E. R. Clore. 1990. Microwave heating of infant formula and breast milk. *J Pediatr Health Care* 4:131-35.
2. Dixon J. J., D. A. Burd, D. G. Roberts. 1997. Severe burns resulting from an exploding teat on a bottle of infant formula milk heated in a microwave oven. *Burns* 23:268-69.

Cleaning and Sanitizing Equipment Used for Bottle Feeding

STANDARD: Bottles, bottle caps, nipples and other equipment used for bottle feeding should not be reused without first being cleaned and sanitized by washing in a dishwasher or by washing, rinsing, and boiling them for one minute.

RATIONALE: Infant feeding bottles are contaminated by the child's saliva during feeding. Formula and milk promote growth of bacteria, yeast, and fungi. Bottles, bottle caps, and nipples that are reused should be washed and sanitized to avoid contamination from previous feedings.

COMMENTS: Excessive boiling of latex bottle nipples will damage them. Nipples that are discolored, thinning, tacky, or ripped should not be used.

Introduction of Age-Appropriate Solid Foods to Infants

STANDARD: A plan to introduce age-appropriate solid foods (complementary foods) to infants should be made in consultation with the child's parent/guardian and primary care provider. Age-appropriate solid foods may be introduced no sooner than when the child has reached the age of four months, but preferably six months and as indicated by the individual child's nutritional and developmental needs.

For breastfed infants, gradual introduction of iron-fortified foods may occur no sooner than around four months, but preferably six months and to complement the human milk. Modification of basic food patterns should be provided in writing by the child's primary care provider.

One new food should be introduced at a time, followed by waiting a couple of days before introducing another new food.

RATIONALE: Early introduction of age-appropriate solid food and fruit juice interferes with the intake of human milk or iron-fortified formula that the infant needs for growth. Age-appropriate solid food given before an infant is developmentally ready may be associated with allergies and digestive problems (1,7). Around about six months of age, breastfed infants may require an additional source of iron. Vitamin drops with iron may be needed. Infants who are not exclusively fed human milk should consume iron-fortified formula as the substitute for human milk (8). In the United States, major non-milk sources of iron in the infant diet are iron-fortified cereal and meats (1). Zinc is important for healthy growth and proper immune function. Infant stores of zinc may subsidize the intake from human milk for several months. Age-appropriate solid foods such as meat (a good source of zinc) are needed beginning at six months (1). A full daily allowance of vitamin C is found in human milk (2). The American Academy of Pediatrics (AAP) recommends that all breastfed or partially breastfed infants receive a minimum daily intake of 400 IU of vitamin D supplementation beginning soon after birth until they consume sufficient vitamin D fortified milk (about one quart per day) to meet the 400 IU daily requirements (3). These supplements should be given at home by the parents/guardians to take the burden off the caregiver/teacher.

The transitional phase of feeding age-appropriate solid foods which occurs no sooner than four months and preferably six months of age is a critical time for development of gross, fine, and oral motor skills. When an infant is able to hold his/her head steady, open her/his mouth, lean forward in anticipation of food offered, close the lips around a spoon, and transfer from front of the tongue to the back and swallow, he/she is ready to eat semi-solid foods. The process of learning a more mature style of eating begins because of physical growth occurring concurrently with social, cultural, sociological, and physiological development.

COMMENTS: Many infants find fruit juices appealing and may be satisfied by the calories in age-appropriate solid foods so that they subsequently drink less human milk or formula. When fruit juice is introduced at one year of age, it should be by cup rather than a bottle or other container (such as a box) to decrease the occurrence of dental caries. Infants, birth up to one year of age, should not be served juice. Whole fruit, mashed or pureed, is appropriate for infants seven months up to one year of age. Children one year of age through age six should be limited to a total of four to six ounces of juice per day.

Many people believe that infants sleep better when they start to eat age-appropriate solid foods, however research shows that longer sleeping periods are developmentally and not nutritionally determined in mid-infancy (1,4).

An important goal of early childhood nutrition is to ensure children's present and future health by fostering the development of healthy eating behaviors (1,8). Caregivers/teachers are responsible for providing a variety of nutritious foods, defining the structure and timing of meals and creating a mealtime environment that facilitates eating and social exchange (6). Children are responsible for participating in choices about food selection and should be allowed to take responsibility for determining how much is consumed at each eating occasion (1).

Good communication between the caregiver/teacher and the parents/guardians cannot be over-emphasized and is essential for successful feeding in general, including when and how to introduce age-appropriate solid foods. The decision to feed specific foods should be made in consultation with the parent/guardian. Caregivers/teachers should be given written instructions on the introduction and feeding of foods from the infant's parent/guardian and primary care provider. Caregivers/teachers can use or develop a take-home sheet for parents/guardians in which the caregiver/teacher records the food consumed, how much, and other important notes on the infant, each day. Caregivers/teachers should continue to consult with each infant's parents/guardians concerning which foods they have introduced and are feeding. This schedule of introducing new foods one at a time with at least a two-day trial period enables parents and caregivers/teachers to pinpoint any problems a child might have with any specific food (9). Following this schedule for introducing new foods, the caregiver/teacher can more easily identify an infant's possible food allergy or intolerance. Consistency between home and the early care and education setting is essential during the period of rapid change when infants are learning to eat age-appropriate solid foods (5,7).

RELATED STANDARDS:

100% Fruit Juice
Written Menus and Introduction of New Foods
Care for Children with Food Allergies
Feeding Age-Appropriate Solid Foods to Infants
Experience with Familiar and New Foods

REFERENCES:

1. Kleinman, R. E., ed. 2009. *Pediatric nutrition handbook*. 6th ed. Elk Grove Village, IL: American Academy of Pediatrics.
2. Lawrence, R. A., R. Lawrence. 2005. *Breast feeding: A guide for the medical profession*. 6th ed. St. Louis: Mosby.
3. Wagner, C. L., F. R. Greer, Section on Breastfeeding, Committee on Nutrition. 2008. Prevention of rickets and vitamin D deficiency in infants, children, and adolescents. *Pediatrics* 122:1142–52.
4. Lally, J. R., A. Griffin, E. Fenichel, M. Segal, E. Szanton, B. Weissbourd. 2003. *Caring for infants and toddlers in groups: Developmentally appropriate practice*. Arlington, VA: Zero to Three.
5. U.S. Department of Agriculture, Food and Nutrition Service. 2002. *Feeding infants: A guide for use in the child nutrition programs*. Rev ed. Alexandria, VA: USDA, FNS. http://www.fns.usda.gov/tn/resources/feeding_infants.pdf.
6. Branscomb, K. R., C. B. Goble. 2008. Infants and toddlers in group care: Feeding practices that foster emotional health. *Young Children* 63:28-33.
7. Grummer-Strawn, L. M., K. S. Scanlon, S. B. Fein. 2008. Infant feeding and feeding transitions during the first year of life. *Pediatrics* 122:S36-42.
8. Griffiths, L. J., L. Smeeth, S. S. Hawkins, T. J. Cole, C. Dezateux. 2008. Effects of infant feeding practice on weight gain from birth to 3 years. *Arch Dis Child* (November): 1-17.
9. Pipes, P. L., C. M. Trahms, eds. 1997. *Nutrition in infancy and childhood*. 6th ed. New York: McGraw-Hill.

Feeding Age-Appropriate Solid Foods to Infants

STANDARD: Staff members should serve commercially packaged baby food from a dish, not directly from a factory-sealed container. They should serve age-appropriate solid food (complementary food) by spoon only. Age-appropriate solid food should not be fed in a bottle or an infant feeder unless written in the child's care plan by the child's primary care provider. Caregivers/teachers should discard uneaten food left in dishes from which they have fed a child. The facility should wash off all jars of baby food with soap and warm water before opening the jars, and examine the food carefully when removing it from the jar to make sure there are not glass pieces or foreign objects in the food.

Food should not be shared among children using the same dish or spoon. Unused portions in opened factory-sealed baby food containers or food brought in containers prepared at home should be stored in the refrigerator and discarded if not consumed after twenty-four hours of storage.

RATIONALE: Feeding of age-appropriate solid foods in a bottle to a child is often associated with premature feeding of age-appropriate solid foods (when the infant is not developmentally ready for them) (1-5).

The external surface of a commercial container may be contaminated with disease-causing microorganisms during shipment or storage and may contaminate the food product during feeding. The portion of the food that is touched by a utensil should be consumed or discarded. A dish should be cleaned and sanitized before use, thereby reducing the likelihood of surface contamination. Any food brought from home should not be served to other children. This will prevent cross-contamination and reinforce the policy that food sent to the facility is for the designated child only.

Uneaten food should not be put back into its original container for storage because it may contain potentially harmful bacteria from the infant's saliva. Age-appropriate solid food should not be fed in a bottle or an infant feeder apparatus because of the potential for choking. Additionally, this feeding method teaches the infant to eat age-appropriate solid foods incorrectly.

RELATED STANDARDS:

Introduction of Age-Appropriate Solid Foods for Infants

REFERENCES:

1. Kleinman, R. E., ed. 2009. *Pediatric nutrition handbook*. 6th ed. Elk Grove Village, IL: American Academy of Pediatrics.
2. Dietitians of Canada, American Dietetic Association. 2000. *Manual of clinical dietetics*. 6th ed. Chicago: ADA.
3. Endres, J. B., R. E. Rockwell. 2003. *Food, nutrition, and the young child*. 4th ed. New York: Macmillan.
4. Samour, P. Q., K. King. 2005. *Handbook of pediatric nutrition*. 3rd ed. Lake Dallas, TX: Helm.
5. Lawrence, R. A., R. Lawrence. 2005. *Breast feeding: A guide for the medical profession*. 6th ed. St. Louis: Mosby.

Use of Soy-Based Formula and Soy Milk

STANDARD: Soy-based formula or soy milk should be provided to a child whose parents/guardians present a written request because of family dietary restrictions on foods produced from animals (i.e. cow's milk and other dairy products). Both soy-based formula and soy milk should be labeled with the infant's or child's full name and date and stored properly.

The caregiver/teacher should collaborate with parents/guardians in exploring community resources to secure soy-based formula. Soy milk should be available for the children of parents/guardians participating in the Women, Infants and Children (WIC) Supplemental Food Program, Child and Adult Care Food Program (CACFP), or Food Stamp Program.

RATIONALE: The American Academy of Pediatrics (AAP) recommends use of hypoallergenic formula (not soy-based formula) for infants who are allergic to cow's milk proteins. Soy-based formulas are appropriate for children with galactosemia or congenital lactose intolerance (1). Because there is a lot of confusion in the public regarding cow's milk proteins and lactose intolerance, these indications should be documented by the child's primary care provider and not based on parental possible misinterpretation of symptoms. Soy-based formulas are made from soy meal (plant based) with added methionine, carbohydrates, and oils (soy or vegetable) and are fortified with vitamins and minerals (2). In the U.S., all soy-based formula is fortified with iron. Soy meal does not contain lactose, so it is used for feeding infants with primary care provider documented congenital lactose intolerance.

COMMENTS: The taste of soy milk is similar to cow's milk. Because soy formula and soy milk are derived from a plant source, parents/guardians may choose these products for dietary (e.g. vegan) or religious reasons. In such cases, soy-based formula is used for infant feeding and unflavored soy milk is the choice for young children.

Caregivers/teachers should encourage parents/guardians of children with primary care provider documented indications for soy formula, participating in WIC and/or Food Stamp Programs, to learn how they can obtain soy-based infant formula or soy milk/products.

Infants may need a variety of special or elemental formulas which are easier to digest and less allergenic.

Elemental or special non-allergic formulas should be specified in the infant's care plan.

RELATED STANDARDS:
Vegetarian/Vegan Diets
Preparing, Feeding, and Storing Infant Formula

REFERENCES:
1. Bhatia, J., F. Greer, Committee on Nutrition. 2008. Use of soy protein-based formulas for infant feeding. *Pediatrics* 121:1062-68.
2. Dietitians of Canada, American Dietetic Association. 2000. *Manual of clinical dietetics*. 6th ed. Chicago: ADA.

Requirements for Toddlers and Preschoolers

Meal and Snack Patterns for Toddlers and Preschoolers

STANDARD: Meals and snacks should contain at least the minimum amount of foods shown in the meal and snack patterns for toddlers and preschoolers described in the Child and Adult Care Food Program (CACFP) guidelines at http://www.fns.usda.gov/cnd/care/ProgramBasics/Meals/Meal_Patterns.htm.

RATIONALE: Even during periods of slower growth, children must continue to eat nutritious foods. With limited appetites and selective eating by toddlers and preschoolers, less nutritious foods should not be served as they can displace more nutritious foods from the child's diet.

COMMENTS: Children who are eating more than one snack and one meal may not want all the food offered at any one of these times. On the other hand, toddlers and preschoolers may eat only some meals or some snacks. The amount of food offered to them must be sufficient to meet their needs at that particular time but not too large to promote overeating.

RELATED STANDARDS:
Categories of Food
Meal and Snack Patterns

Serving Size for Toddlers and Preschoolers

STANDARD: The facility should serve toddlers and preschoolers small-sized, age-appropriate portions and should permit children to have one or more additional servings of the nutritious foods that are low in fat, sugar, and sodium as needed to meet the caloric needs of the individual child. Serving dishes should contain the appropriate amount of food based on serving sizes or portions recommended for each child and adult as described in the Child and Adult Care Food Program (CACFP) guidelines at http://www.fns.usda.gov/cnd/care/ProgramBasics/Meals/Meal_Patterns.htm. Young children should learn what appropriate portion size is by being served in plates, bowls, and cups that are developmentally appropriate to their nutritional needs.

Food service staff and/or a caregiver/teacher is responsible for preparing the amount of food based on the recommended age-appropriate amount of food per serving for each child to be fed. Usually a reasonable amount of additional food is prepared to respond to a child or children requesting a second serving of the nutritious foods that are low in fat, sugar, and sodium.

RATIONALE: Gradual extension of the diet begun in infancy should continue throughout the preschool period. A child will not eat the same amount each day because appetites vary and food sprees are common (1-5). If normal variations in eating patterns are accepted without comment, feeding problems usually do not develop. Requiring that a child eat a specified food or amount of food may be counterproductive. Eating habits established in infancy and early childhood may contribute to suboptimal eating patterns later in life. Including nutritious snacks in the daily meal plan will help to ensure that the child's nutrient needs are met. The quality of snacks for young children and school-age children is especially important, and small, frequent feedings are recommended to achieve the total desired daily intake.

Strong evidence supports that larger plate, bowl, and cup sizes promote overeating in adults (6,7). It is likely that the same is true in children. Larger serving sizes and what is considered "normal" serving size (portion size distortion), at least in part is explained by increasing size of plates, bowls, and cups.

COMMENTS: Continuing to meet the child's needs for growth and activity is important. During the second and third years of life, the child grows much less rapidly than during the first year of life.

Standardized recipes for cooking for young children are available and are a valuable resource. Periodic training is also available from resources such as regional Head Start agencies, State Child Care agencies, resource and referral agencies, local health departments, local colleges, and universities.

Size appropriate plates, bowls, and cups in early care and education settings should help children and caregivers/teachers recognize and understand appropriate portion sizes. They may also help decrease the risk of overeating.

RELATED STANDARDS:
Meal and Snack Patterns for Toddlers and Preschoolers
Encouraging Self-Feeding by Older Infants and Toddlers

REFERENCES:
1. Kleinman, R. E., ed. 2009. *Pediatric nutrition handbook*. 6th ed. Elk Grove Village, IL: American Academy of Pediatrics.
2. Endres, J. B., R. E. Rockwell. 2003. *Food, nutrition, and the young child*. 4th ed. New York: Macmillan.
3. U.S. Department of Agriculture, Food Service and Nutrition. 2009. Child and adult care food program. http://www.fns.usda.gov/CND/Care/CACFP/aboutcacfp.htm.
4. U.S. Department of Agriculture. 2002. *Making nutrition count for children – Nutrition guidance for child care homes*. Washington, DC: USDA.
5. Pipes, P. L., C. M. Trahms, eds. 1997. *Nutrition in infancy and childhood*. 6th ed. New York: McGraw-Hill.
6. Wansink, B. 2004. Environmental factors that increase the food intake and consumption volume of unknowing consumers. *Annual Review of Nutrition* 24:455-79.
7. Wansink, B., J. E. Painter, J. North. 2005. Bottomless bowls: Why visual cues of portion size may influence intake. *Obesity Research* 13:93-100.

Encouraging Self-Feeding by Older Infants and Toddlers

STANDARD: Caregivers/teachers should encourage older infants and toddlers to hold and drink from an appropriate child-sized cup, to use a child-sized spoon (short handle with a shallow bowl like a soup spoon), a child-sized fork (short, blunt tines and broad handle similar to a salad fork), all of which are developmentally appropriate for young children to feed themselves, and to use their fingers for self-feeding.

RATIONALE: As children enter the second year of life, they are interested in doing things for themselves. Self-feeding appropriately separates the responsibilities of adults and children. The adult is responsible for providing nutritious food, and the child is responsible for deciding how much of it to eat (1-5). To allow for the proper development of motor skills and eating habits, children need to be allowed to practice learning to feed themselves (6-8). Children in group care should be provided with opportunities to serve and eat a variety of food for themselves. Children will continue to self-feed using their fingers even after mastering the use of a utensil.

COMMENTS: Foods served should be appropriate to the toddler's developmental ability and cut small enough to avoid choking hazards.

RELATED STANDARDS:
Serving Size for Toddlers and Preschoolers
Numbers of Children Fed Simultaneously by One Adult
Adult Supervision of Children Who are Learning to Feed Themselves

REFERENCES:
1. Benjamin, S. E., ed. 2007. *Making food healthy and safe for children: How to meet the national health and safety performance standards – Guidelines for out of home child care programs*. 2nd ed. Chapel Hill, NC: National Training Institute for Child Care Health Consultants. http://nti.unc.edu/course_files/curriculum/nutrition/making_food_healthy_and_safe.pdf.
2. Kleinman, R. E., ed. 2009. *Pediatric nutrition handbook*. 6th ed. Elk Grove Village, IL: American Academy of Pediatrics.
3. Endres, J. B., R. E. Rockwell. 2003. *Food, nutrition, and the young child*. 4th ed. New York: Macmillan.
4. Pipes, P. L., C. M. Trahms, eds. 1997. *Nutrition in infancy and childhood*. 6th ed. New York: McGraw-Hill.
5. Briley, M. E., C. Roberts-Gray. 1999. Position of the American Dietetic Association: Nutrition standards for child-care programs. *J Am Diet Assoc* 99:981-88.
6. Branscomb, K. R., C. B. Goble. 2008. Infants and toddlers in group care: Feeding practices that foster emotional health. *Young Children* 63:28-33.
7. Hagan, J. F., J. S. Shaw, P. M. Duncan, eds. 2008. *Bright futures: Guidelines for health supervision of infants, children, and adolescents*. 3rd ed. Elk Grove Village, IL: American Academy of Pediatrics.
8. University of Idaho, College of Agricultural and Life Sciences. *Feeding young children in group settings*. http://www.cals.uidaho.edu/feeding/.

Feeding Cow's Milk

STANDARD: The facility should not serve cow's milk to infants from birth to twelve months of age, unless provided with a written exception and direction from the child's primary care provider and parents/guardians. Children between twelve and twenty-four months of age, who are not on human milk or prescribed formula, can be served whole pasteurized milk, or reduced fat (2%) pasteurized milk for those children who are at risk for hypercholesterolemia or obesity (1). Children two years of age and older should be served skim or 1% pasteurized milk.

RATIONALE: For children between twelve months and twenty-four months of age, for whom overweight or obesity is a concern or who have a family history of obesity, dyslipidemia, or early cardiovascular disease, the use of reduced fat (2%) milk is appropriate (1). The child's primary care provider may also recommend reduced fat (2%) milk for some children this age. Studies show no compromise in growth, and no difference in height, weight, or percentage of body fat and neurological development in toddlers fed reduced fat (2%) milk compared with those fed whole milk (2,8,9). The American Academy of Pediatrics recommends that cow's milk not be used during the first year of life (3-7).

COMMENTS: Sometimes early care and education programs have children ages eighteen months to three years of age in one classroom and staff report it is difficult to serve different types of milk (1% and 2%) to specific children. Programs can use a different color label for each type of milk on the container or pitcher. Caregivers/teachers can explain to the children the meaning of the color labels and identify which milk they are drinking.

RELATED STANDARDS:
Categories of Foods

REFERENCES:

1. Daniels, S. R., F. R. Greer, Committee on Nutrition. 2008. Lipid screening and cardiovascular health in childhood. *Pediatrics* 122:198-208.
2. Wosje, K. S., B. L. Specker, J. Giddens. 2001. No differences in growth or body composition from age 12 to 24 months between toddlers consuming 2% milk and toddlers consuming whole milk. *J Am Diet Assoc* 101:53-56.
3. Dietz, W. H., L. Stern, eds. 1998. *American Academy of Pediatrics guide to your child's nutrition*. New York: Villard.
4. Kleinman, R. E., ed. 2009. *Pediatric nutrition handbook*. 6th ed. Elk Grove Village, IL: American Academy of Pediatrics.
5. Dietitians of Canada, American Dietetic Association. 2000. *Manual of clinical dietetics*. 6th ed. Chicago: ADA.
6. Pipes, P. L., C. M. Trahms, eds. 1997. *Nutrition in infancy and childhood*. 6th ed. New York: McGraw-Hill.
7. American Academy of Pediatrics, Committee on Nutrition. 1992. The use of whole cow's milk in infancy. *Pediatrics* 89:1105-9.
8. Rask-Nissila, L., E. Jokinen, P. Terho, A. Tammi, H. Lapinleimu, T. Ronnemaa, J. Viikari, R. Seppanen, T. Korhonen, J. Tuominen, I. Valimaki, O. Simell. 2000. Neurological development of 5-year-old children receiving a low-saturated fat, low-cholesterol diet since infancy: A randomized controlled trial. *JAMA* 284:993-1000.
9. Niinikoski, H. Lapinleimu, , J. Viikari, H. Lapinleimu, T. Rönnemaa, E. Jokinen, R. Seppänen, P. Terho, J. Tuominen, I. Välimäki, O. Simell. 1997. Growth until 3 years of age in a prospective, randomized trial of a diet with reduced saturated fat and cholesterol. *Pediatrics* 99:687-94.

Requirements for School-Age Children

Meal and Snack Patterns for School-Age Children

STANDARD: Meals and snacks should contain at a minimum the meal and snack patterns shown for school-age children in the Child and Adult Care Food Program (CACFP) guidelines found at http://www.fns.usda.gov/cnd/care/ProgramBasics/Meals/Meal_Patterns.htm.

Children attending facilities for two or more hours after school need at least one snack.

Breakfast is recommended for all children enrolled in an early care and education facility or in school. Depending on age, in-between eating such as a snack should occur about two hours after a meal based on the total length of time a child is in care. Child care facilities enrolled in the CACFP must allow at least one and a half hours between the end of a snack and the beginning of another meal and they must allow three hours between the end of one meal to the beginning of the next meal. CACFP requirements differ from state to state, see CACFP's Website for current recommendations.

RATIONALE: The principles of providing adequate, nourishing food for younger children apply to this group as well. This age is characterized by a rapid rate of growth that increases the need for energy and essential nutrients to support optimal growth. Food intake may vary considerably because this is a time when children express strong food likes and dislikes. The quantity and quality of food provided should contribute toward meeting nutritional needs for the day and should not dull the appetite (1-5).

COMMENTS: A nutrient analysis was conducted of the CACFP requirements, to ensure that a snack and lunch meet two-thirds of the Recommended Dietary Allowances (6).

REFERENCES:

1. Hagan, J. F., J. S. Shaw, P. M. Duncan, eds. 2008. *Bright futures: Guidelines for health supervision of infants, children, and adolescents*. 3rd ed. Elk Grove Village, IL: American Academy of Pediatrics.
2. Story, M., K. Holt, D. Sofka, eds. 2002. *Bright futures in practice: Nutrition*. 2nd ed. Arlington, VA: National Center for Education in Maternal and Child Health. http://www.brightfutures.org/nutrition/pdf/frnt_mttr.pdf.
3. Benjamin, S. E., ed. 2007. *Making food healthy and safe for children: How to meet the national health and safety performance standards – Guidelines*

for out of home child care programs. 2nd ed. Chapel Hill, NC: National Training Institute for Child Care Health Consultants. http://nti.unc.edu/course_files/curriculum/nutrition/making_food_healthy_and_safe.pdf.
4. Endres, J. B., R. E. Rockwell. 2003. *Food, nutrition, and the young child*. 4th ed. New York: Macmillan.
5. Pipes, P. L., C. M. Trahms, eds. 1997. *Nutrition in infancy and childhood*. 6th ed. New York: McGraw-Hill.
6. Briley, M. E., C. Roberts-Gray. 1999. Position of the American Dietetic Association: Nutrition standards for child-care programs. *J Am Diet Assoc* 99:981-88.

Meal Service and Supervision

Socialization During Meals

STANDARD: Caregivers/teachers and children should sit at the table and eat the meal or snack together. Family style meal service, with the serving platters, bowls, and pitchers on the table so all present can serve themselves, should be encouraged, except for infants and very young children who require an adult to feed them. A separate utensil should be used for serving. Children should not handle foods that they will not be consuming. The adults should encourage, but not force, the children to help themselves to all food components offered at the meal. When eating meals with children, the adult(s) should eat items that meet nutrition standards. The adult(s) should encourage social interaction and conversation, using vocabulary related to the concepts of color, shape, size, quantity, number, temperature of food, and events of the day. Extra assistance and time should be provided for slow eaters. Eating should be an enjoyable experience at the facility and at home.

Special accommodations should be made for children who cannot have the food that is being served. Children who need limited portion sizes should be taught and monitored.

RATIONALE: "Family style" meal service promotes and supports social, emotional, and gross and fine motor skill development. Caregivers/teachers sitting and eating with children is an opportunity to engage children in social interactions with each other and for positive role-modeling by the adult caregiver/teacher. Conversation at the table adds to the pleasant mealtime environment and provides opportunities for informal modeling of appropriate eating behaviors, communication about eating, and imparting nutrition learning experiences (1-3,5-7). The presence of an adult or adults, who eat with the children, helps prevent behaviors that increase the possibility of fighting, feeding each other, stuffing food into the mouth and potential choking, and other negative behaviors. The future development of children depends, to no small extent, on their command of language. Richness of language increases as adults and peers nurture it (5). Family style meals encourage children to serve themselves which develops their eye-hand coordination (3-5). In addition to being nourished by food, infants and young children are encouraged to establish warm human relationships by their eating experiences. When children lack the developmental skills for self-feeding, they will be unable to serve food to themselves. An adult seated at the table can assist and be supportive with self-feeding so the child can eat an adequate amount of food to promote growth and prevent hunger.

COMMENTS: Compliance is measured by structured observation. Use of small pitchers, a limited number of portions on service plates, and adult assistance to enable children to successfully serve themselves helps to make family style service possible without contamination or waste of food.

RELATED STANDARDS:
Encouraging Self-Feeding by Older Infants and Toddlers
Serving Size for Toddlers and Preschoolers
Nutrition Learning Experiences for Children

REFERENCES:
1. U.S. Department of Health and Human Services, Administration for Children and Families, Office of Head Start. 2009. *Head Start program performance standards*. Rev. ed. Washington, DC: U.S. Government Printing Office. http://eclkc.ohs.acf.hhs.gov/hslc/Program%20Design%20and%20Management/Head%20Start%20Requirements/Head%20Start%20Requirements/45%20CFR%20Chapter%20XIII/45%20CFR%20Chap%20XIII_ENG.pdf.
2. Benjamin, S. E., ed. 2007. *Making food healthy and safe for children: How to meet the national health and safety performance standards – Guidelines for out of home child care programs*. 2nd ed. Chapel Hill, NC: National Training Institute for Child Care Health Consultants. http://nti.unc.edu/course_files/curriculum/nutrition/making_food_healthy_and_safe.pdf.
3. Endres, J. B., R. E. Rockwell. 2003. *Food, nutrition, and the young child*. 4th ed. New York: Macmillan.
4. U.S. Department of Agriculture. 2002. *Making nutrition count for children - Nutrition guidance for child care homes*. Washington, DC: USDA.
5. Pipes, P. L., C. M. Trahms, eds. 1997. *Nutrition in infancy and childhood*. 6th ed. New York: McGraw-Hill.
6. Branscomb, K. R., C. B. Goble 2008. Infants and toddlers in group care: Feeding practices that foster emotional health. *Young Children* 63:28-33.
7. Sigman-Grant, M., E. Christiansen, L. Branen, J. Fletcher, S. L. Johnson. 2008. About feeding children: Mealtimes in child-care centers in four western states. *J Am Diet Assoc* 108:340-46.

Numbers of Children Fed Simultaneously by One Adult

STANDARD: One adult should not feed more than one infant or three children who need adult assistance with feeding at the same time.

RATIONALE: Cross-contamination among children whom one adult is feeding simultaneously poses significant risk. In addition, mealtime should be a socializing occasion. Feeding more than three children at the same time necessarily resembles an impersonal production line. It is difficult for the caregiver/teacher to be aware of and respond to infant feeding cues when feeding more than one infant at a time. A child may need one-on-one feeding based on age or degree of ability. Feeding more than three children also presents a potential risk of injury and/or choking.

RELATED STANDARDS:
Feeding Infants on Cue by a Consistent Caregiver/Teacher
Encouraging Self-Feeding by Older Infants and Toddlers
Serving Size for Toddlers and Preschoolers
Socialization During Meals
Adult Supervision of Children Who are Learning to Feed Themselves

Adult Supervision of Children Who are Learning to Feed Themselves

STANDARD: Children in mid-infancy who are learning to feed themselves should be supervised by an adult seated within arm's reach of them at all times while they are being fed. Children over twelve months of age who can feed themselves should be supervised by an adult who is seated at the same table or within arm's reach of the child's highchair or feeding table. When eating, children should be within sight of an adult at all times.

RATIONALE: A supervising adult should watch for several common problems that typically occur when children in mid-infancy begin to feed themselves. "Squirreling" of several pieces of food in the mouth increases the likelihood of choking. A choking child may not make any noise, so adults must keep their eyes on children who are eating. Active supervision is imperative. Supervised eating also promotes the child's safety by discouraging activities that can lead to choking (1). For best practice, children of all ages should be supervised when eating. Adults can monitor age-appropriate portion size consumption.

COMMENTS: Adults can help children while they are learning, by modeling active chewing (i.e., eating a small piece of food, showing how to use their teeth to bite it) and making positive comments to encourage children while they are eating. Adults can demonstrate how to eat foods on the menu, how to serve food, and how to ask for more food as a way of helping children learn the names of foods (i.e. "please pass the bowl of noodles").

RELATED STANDARDS:
Encouraging Self-Feeding by Older Infants and Toddlers
Socialization During Meals
Numbers of Children Fed Simultaneously by One Adult

REFERENCES:
1. American Academy of Pediatrics, Committee on Injury, Violence, and Poison Prevention. 2010. Policy statement: Prevention of choking among children. *Pediatrics* 125:601-7

Participation of Older Children and Staff in Mealtime Activities

STANDARD: Both older children and staff should be actively involved in serving food and other mealtime activities, such as setting and cleaning the table. Staff should supervise and assist children with appropriate handwashing procedures before and after meals and sanitizing of eating surfaces and utensils to prevent cross contamination.

RATIONALE: Children develop social skills and new motor skills as well as increase their dexterity through this type of involvement. Children require close supervision by staff and other adults when they use knives and have contact with food surfaces and food that other children will use.

COMMENTS: Compliance is measured by structured observation.

RELATED STANDARDS:
Socialization During Meals

Experience with Familiar and New Foods

STANDARD: In consultation with the family and the Nutritionist/Registered Dietitian, caregivers/teachers should offer children familiar foods that are typical of the child's culture and religious preferences and should also introduce a variety of healthful foods that may not be familiar, but meet a child's nutritional needs. Experiences with new foods can include tasting and swallowing but also include engagement of all senses (seeing, smelling, speaking, etc.) to facilitate the introduction of these new foods.

RATIONALE: By learning about new food, children increase their knowledge of the world around them, and the likelihood that they will choose a more varied, better balanced diet in later life. Eating habits and attitudes about food formed in the early years often last a lifetime. New food acceptance may take eight to fifteen times of offering a food before it is eaten (1).

RELATED STANDARDS:
Written Menus and Introduction of New Foods
Introduction of Age-Appropriate Solid Foods to Infants

REFERENCES:
1. Sullivan, S. A., L. L. Birch. 1990. Pass the sugar, pass the salt: Experience dictates preference. *Developmental Psychology* 26:546-51.

Activities that are Incompatible with Eating

STANDARD: Children should be seated when eating. Caregivers/teachers should ensure that children do not eat when standing, walking, running, playing, lying down, watching TV, playing on the computer, or riding in vehicles.

Children should not be allowed to continue to feed themselves or continue to be assisted with feeding themselves if they begin to fall asleep while eating. Caregivers/teachers should check that no food is left in a child's mouth before laying a child down to sleep.

RATIONALE: Seating children, while they are eating, reduces the risk of aspiration (1-4). Eating while doing other activities (including playing, walking around, or sitting at a computer) limits opportunities for socialization during meals and snacks. Eating while watching television is associated with an increased risk of obesity (5-8). Continuing to eat while falling asleep puts the child at great risk for gagging or choking.

COMMENTS: Staff can role model appropriate eating behaviors by sitting down when they are eating and eating "family style" with the children when possible.

RELATED STANDARDS:
Socialization During Meals

REFERENCES:
1. Benjamin, S. E., ed. 2007. *Making food healthy and safe for children: How to meet the national health and safety performance standards – Guidelines for out of home child care programs.* 2nd ed. Chapel Hill, NC: National Training Institute for Child Care Health Consultants. http://nti.unc.edu/course_files/curriculum/nutrition/making_food_healthy_and_safe.pdf.
2. Lally, J. R., A. Griffin, E. Fenichel, M. Segal, E. Szanton, B. Weissbourd. 2003. *Caring for infants and toddlers in groups: Developmentally appropriate practice.* Arlington, VA: Zero to Three.
3. Endres, J. B., R. E. Rockwell. 2003. *Food, nutrition, and the young child.* 4th ed. New York: Macmillan.
4. U.S. Department of Agriculture. 2002. *Making nutrition count for children - Nutrition guidance for child care homes.* Washington, DC: USDA.
5. Briley, M., C. Roberts-Gray. 2005. Position of the American Dietetic Association: Benchmarks for nutrition programs in child care settings. *J Am Dietetic Association* 105:979–86.
6. Andersen, R. E., C. J. Crespo, S. J. Bartlett, L. J. Cheskin, M. Pratt. 1998. Relationship of physical activity and television watching with body weight and level of fatness among children. *J Am Med Assoc* 279:938-42.
7. Dennison, B. A., T. A. Erb, P. L. Jenkins. 2002. Television viewing and television in bedroom associated with overweight risk among low-income preschool children. *Pediatrics* 109:1028-35.
8. Mendoza, J. A., F. J. Zimmerman, D. A. Christakis. 2007. Television viewing, computer use, obesity, and adiposity in US preschool children. *Int J Behav Nutr and Physical Activity* 4, no. 44 (September 25). http://ijbnpa.org/content/4/1/44.

Prohibited Uses of Food

STANDARD: Caregivers/teachers should not force or bribe children to eat nor use food as a reward or punishment.

RATIONALE: Children who are forced to eat or, for whom adults use food to modify behavior, come to view eating as a tug-of-war and are more likely to develop lasting food dislikes and unhealthy eating behaviors. Offering food as a reward or punishment places undue importance on food and may have negative effects on the child by promoting "clean the plate" responses that may lead to obesity or poor eating behavior (1-5).

COMMENTS: All components of the meal should be offered at the same time, allowing children to select and enjoy all of the foods on the menu.

REFERENCES:

1. U.S. Department of Health and Human Services, Administration for Children and Families, Office of Head Start. 2009. *Head Start program performance standards*. Rev. ed. Washington, DC: U.S. Government Printing Office. http://eclkc.ohs.acf.hhs.gov/hslc/Program%20Design%20and%20Management/Head%20Start%20Requirements/Head%20Start%20Requirements/45%20CFR%20Chapter%20XIII/45%20CFR%20Chap%20XIII_ENG.pdf.
2. Kleinman, R. E., ed. 2009. *Pediatric nutrition handbook*. 6th ed. Elk Grove Village, IL: American Academy of Pediatrics.
3. Murph, J. R., S. D. Palmer, D. Glassy, eds. 2005. *Health in child care: A manual for health professionals*. Elk Grove Village, IL: American Academy of Pediatrics.
4. Benjamin, S. E., ed. 2007. *Making food healthy and safe for children: How to meet the national health and safety performance standards – Guidelines for out of home child care programs*. 2nd ed. Chapel Hill, NC: National Training Institute for Child Care Health Consultants. http://nti.unc.edu/course_files/curriculum/nutrition/making_food_healthy_and_safe.pdf.
5. Birch, L. L., J. O. Fisher, K. K. Davison. 2003. Learning to overeat: Maternal use of restrictive feeding practices promotes girls' eating in the absence of hunger. *Am J Clin Nutr* 78:215-20.

Use of Nutritionist/Registered Dietitian

STANDARD: A local Nutritionist/Registered Dietitian knowledgeable of the specific needs of infants and children, should work with the on-site food service expert and the architect or engineer on the design of the parts of the facility involved in food service. Additionally the Nutritionist/Registered Dietitian should work with the food service expert and the early care and education staff to develop and to implement the facility's nutrition plan and to prepare the initial food service budget. The nutrition plan encompasses:

a. Kitchen layout;
b. Food budget and service;
c. Food procurement and food storage;
d. Menu and meal planning (including periodic review of menus);
e. Food preparation and service;
f. Child feeding practices and policies;
g. Kitchen and mealtime staffing;
h. Nutrition education for children, staff and parents/guardians (including the prevention of childhood obesity and other chronic diseases, food learning experiences, and knowledge of choking hazards);
i. Dietary modification plans

RATIONALE: Efficient and cost-effective food service in a facility begins with a plan and evaluation of the physical components of the facility. Planning for the food service unit includes consideration of location and adequacy of space for receiving, storing, preparing, and serving areas; cleaning up; dish washing; dining areas, plus space for desk, telephone, records, and employee facilities (such as handwashing sinks, toilets, and lockers). All facets must be considered for new or existing sites, including remodeling or renovation of the unit (1-5).

COMMENTS: Nutritionists/Registered Dietitians assist food service staff/caregivers/teachers in planning menus for meals/snacks consisting of healthy foods which meet CACFP guidelines; ensuring use of age appropriate eating utensils and suitable furniture (tables, chairs) for children to sit comfortably while eating; addressing any dietary modification needed; providing training for staff and nutrition education for children and their parents/guardians; consulting on meeting local health department regulations and meeting local regulations when using an off-site food vendor. This standard is primarily for Centers.

RELATED STANDARDS:

Written Nutrition Plan
Routine Health Supervision and Growth Monitoring
Assessment and Planning of Nutrition for Individual Children
Feeding Plans and Dietary Modifications
Food and Nutrition Service Policies and Plans
Appendix – Nutritionist/Registered Dietitian, Consultant and Food Service Staff Qualifications

REFERENCES:

1. Endres, J. B., R. E. Rockwell. 2003. *Food, nutrition, and the young child*. 4th ed. New York: Macmillan.
2. U.S. Department of Agriculture. 2002. *Making nutrition count for children - Nutrition guidance for child care homes*. Washington, DC: USDA.
3. Pipes, P. L., C. M. Trahms, eds. 1997. Nutrition in infancy and childhood. 6th ed. New York: McGraw-Hill.
4. Benjamin, S. E., K. A. Copeland, A. Cradock, E. Walker, M. M. Slining, B. Neelon, M. W. Gillman. 2009. Menus in child care: A comparison of state regulations to national standards. *J Am Diet Assoc* 109:109-15.
5. Kaphingst, K. M., M. Story. 2009. Child care as an untapped setting for obesity prevention: State child care licensing regulations related to nutrition, physical activity, and media use for preschool-aged children in the United States. *Prev Chronic Dis* 6(1).

Food Brought from Home

Nutritional Quality of Food Brought from Home

STANDARD: The facility should provide parents/guardians with written guidelines that the facility has established a comprehensive plan to meet the nutritional requirements of the children in the facility's care and suggested ways parents/guardians can assist the facility in meeting these guidelines. The facility should develop policies for foods brought from home, with parent/guardian consultation, so that expectations are the same for all families (1,2). The facility should have food available to supplement a child's food brought from home if the food brought from home is deficient in meeting the child's nutrient requirements. If the food the parent/guardian provides consistently does not meet the nutritional or food safety requirements, the facility should provide the food and refer the parent/guardian for consultation to a Nutritionist/Registered Dietitian, to the child's primary care provider, or to community resources with trained nutritionists/registered dietitians (such as The Women, Infants and Children [WIC] Supplemental Food Program, extension services, and health departments).

RATIONALE: The caregiver/teacher/facility has a responsibility to follow feeding practices that promote optimum nutrition supporting growth and development in infants, toddlers, and children. Caregivers/teachers who fail to follow best feeding practices, even when parents/guardians wish such counter practices to be followed, negate their basic responsibility of protecting a child's health, social, and emotional well being.

COMMENTS: Some local health and/or licensing jurisdictions prohibit any foods being brought from home.

RELATED STANDARDS:
Written Nutrition Plan
Selection and Preparation of Food Brought from Home
Food and Nutrition Service Policies and Plans

REFERENCES:
1. Sweitzer, S., M. E. Briley, C. Robert-Gray. 2009. Do sack lunches provided by parents meet the nutritional needs of young children who attend child care? *J Am Diet Assn* 109:141-44.
2. Contra Costa Child Care Council, Child Health and Nutrition Program. *CHOICE: Creating healthy opportunities in child care environments.* Concord, CA: Contra Costa Child Care Council, Child Health and Nutrition Program. http://w2.cocokids.org/_cs/downloadables/cc-healthnutrition-choicetoolkit.pdf.

Selection and Preparation of Food Brought from Home

STANDARD: The parent/guardian may provide meals for the child upon written agreement between the parent/guardian and the staff. Food brought into the facility should have a clear label showing the child's full name, the date, and the type of food. Lunches and snacks the parent/guardian provides for one individual child's meals should not be shared with other children. When foods are brought to the facility from home or elsewhere, these foods should be limited to those listed in the facility's written policy on nutritional quality of food brought from home. Potentially hazardous and perishable foods should be refrigerated and all foods should be protected against contamination.

RATIONALE: Food borne illness and poisoning from food is a common occurrence when food has not been properly refrigerated and covered. Although many such illnesses are limited to vomiting and diarrhea, sometimes they are life-threatening. Restricting food sent to the facility to be consumed by the individual child reduces the risk of food poisoning from unknown procedures used in home preparation, storage, and transport. Food brought from home should be nourishing, clean, and safe for an individual child. In this way, other children should not be exposed to unknown risk. Inadvertent sharing of food is a common occurrence in early care and education. The facility has an obligation to ensure that any food offered to children at the facility or shared with other children is wholesome and safe as well as complying with the food and nutrition guidelines for meals and snacks that the early care and education program should observe.

COMMENTS: The facility, in collaboration with parents and the Food Service Staff/Nutritionist/Registered Dietitian, should establish a policy on foods brought from home for celebrating a child's birthday or any similar festive occasion. Programs should inform parents/guardians about healthy food alternatives like fresh fruit cups or fruit salad for such celebrations. Sweetened treats are highly discouraged, but if provided by the parent/guardian, then the portion size of the treat served should be small.

RELATED STANDARDS:
Nutritional Quality of Food Brought from Home
Food and Nutrition Service Policies and Plans

Nutrition Education

Nutrition Learning Experiences for Children

STANDARD: The facility should have a nutrition plan that integrates the introduction of food and feeding experiences with facility activities and home feeding. The plan should include opportunities for children to develop the knowledge and skills necessary to make appropriate food choices.

For centers, this plan should be a written plan and should be the shared responsibility of the entire staff, including directors and food service personnel, together with parents/guardians. The nutrition plan should be developed with guidance from, and should be approved by, the Nutritionist/Registered Dietitian or Child Care Health Consultant.

Caregivers/teachers should teach children about the taste, smell, texture of foods, and vocabulary and language skills related to food and eating. The children should have the opportunity to feel the textures and learn the different colors, sizes, and shapes of foods and the nutritional benefits of eating healthy foods. Children should also be taught about appropriate portion sizes. The teaching should be evident at mealtimes and during curricular activities, and emphasize the pleasure of eating. Caregivers/teachers need to be aware that children between the ages of two- and five-years-old are often resistant to trying new foods and that food acceptance may take eight to fifteen times of offering a food before it is eaten (14).

RATIONALE: Nourishing and attractive food is a foundation for developmentally appropriate learning experiences and contributes to health and well-being (1-13,15). Coordinating the learning experiences with the food service staff maximizes effectiveness of the education. In addition to the nutritive value of food, infants and young children are helped, through the act of feeding, to establish warm human relationships. Eating should be an enjoyable experience for children and staff in the facility and for children and parents/guardians at home. Enjoying and learning about food in childhood promotes good nutrition habits for a lifetime (17,18).

COMMENTS: Parents/guardians and caregivers/teachers should always be encouraged to sit at the table and eat the same food offered to young children as a way to strengthen family style eating which supports child's serving and feeding him or herself (19). Family style eating requires special training for the food service and early care and education staff since they need to monitor food served in a group setting. Portions should be age-appropriate as specified in Child and Adult Care Food Program (CACFP) guidelines. The use of serving utensils should be encouraged to minimize food handling by children. Children should not eat directly out of serving dishes or storage containers. The presence of an adult at the table with children while they are eating is a way to encourage social interaction and conversation about the food such as its name, color, texture, taste, and concepts such as number, size, and shape; as well as sharing events of the day. These are some practical examples of age-appropriate information for young children to learn about the food they eat. The parent/guardian or adult can help the slow eater, prevent behaviors that might increase risk of fighting, of eating each others' food, and of stuffing food in the mouth in such a way that it might cause choking.

Several community-based nutrition resources can help caregivers/teachers with the nutrition and food service component of their programs (16,17,18). The key to identifying a qualified nutrition professional is seeking a record of training in pediatric nutrition (normal nutrition, nutrition for children with special health care needs, dietary modifications) and experience and competency in basic food service systems.

Local resources for nutrition education include:

- Local and state nutritionists in health departments, in maternal and child health programs, and divisions of children with special health care needs;
- Nutritionists/Registered Dietitians at hospitals;
- The Women, Infants, and Children (WIC) Supplemental Food Program and cooperative extension nutritionists;
- School food service personnel;
- State administrators of the Child and Adult Care Food Program;
- National School Food Service Management Institute;
- Healthy Meals Resource System of the Food and Nutrition Information System (National Agricultural Library, U.S. Department of Agriculture);
- Nutrition consultants with local affiliates of the following organizations:
  - o American Dietetic Association;

- o American Public Health Association;
- o Society for Nutrition Education;
- o American Association of Family and Consumer Sciences;
- o Dairy Council;
- o American Heart Association;
- o American Cancer Society;
- o American Diabetes Association;
- o Professional home economists like teachers and those with consumer organizations;
- o Nutrition departments of local colleges and universities.

Compliance is measured by structured observation.

Following are select resources for caregivers in providing ongoing opportunities for children and their families to learn about food and healthy eating.

- Brieger, K. M. 1993. *Cooking up the Pyramid: An early childhood nutrition curriculum*. Pine Island, NY: Clinical Nutrition Services.
- Cunningham, M. 1995. *Cooking with children: 15 lessons for children, age 7 and up, who really want to learn to cook*. New York: Alfred A. Knopf.
- Goodwin, M. T., G. Pollen. 1980. *Creative food experiences for children*. Rev. ed. Washington, DC: Center for Science in the Public Interest.
- King, M. 1993. *Healthy choices for kids: Nutrition and activity education program based on the US Dietary Guidelines. Levels 1-3 and 4-5*. Wenatchee, WA: The Growers of Washington State Apples.

RELATED STANDARDS:

Written Nutrition Plan
Socialization During Meals
Participation of Older Children and Staff in Mealtime Activities
Experience with Familiar and New Foods
Health, Nutrition, Physical Activity, and Safety Awareness
Nutrition Education for Parents/Guardians
Food and Nutrition Service Policies and Plans
Appendix – Nutritionist/Registered Dietitian, Consultant, and Food Service Staff Qualifications

REFERENCES:

1. U.S. Department of Health and Human Services, Administration for Children and Families, Office of Head Start. 2009. *Head Start program performance standards*. Rev. ed. Washington, DC: U.S. Government Printing Office. http://eclkc.ohs.acf.hhs.gov/hslc/Program%20Design%20and%20Management/Head%20Start%20Requirements/Head%20Start%20Requirements/45%20CFR%20Chapter%20XIII/45%20CFR%20Chap%20XIII_ENG.pdf.
2. Hagan, J. F., J. S. Shaw, P. M. Duncan, eds. 2008. *Bright futures: Guidelines for health supervision of infants, children, and adolescents*. 3rd ed. Elk Grove Village, IL: American Academy of Pediatrics.
3. Story, M., K. Holt, D. Sofka, eds. 2002. *Bright futures in practice: Nutrition*. 2nd ed. Arlington, VA: National Center for Education in Maternal and Child Health. http://www.brightfutures.org/nutrition/pdf/frnt_mttr.pdf.
4. Wardle, F., N. Winegarner. 1992. Nutrition and Head Start. *Child Today* 21:57.
5. Benjamin, S. E., ed. 2007. *Making food healthy and safe for children: How to meet the national health and safety performance standards – Guidelines for out of home child care programs*. 2nd ed. Chapel Hill, NC: National Training Institute for Child Care Health Consultants. http://nti.unc.edu/course_files/curriculum/nutrition/making_food_healthy_and_safe.pdf.
6. Dietz, W. H., L. Stern, eds. 1998. *American Academy of Pediatrics guide to your child's nutrition*. New York: Villard.
7. Kleinman, R. E., ed. 2009. *Pediatric nutrition handbook*. 6th ed. Elk Grove Village, IL: American Academy of Pediatrics.
8. Lally, J. R., A. Griffin, E. Fenichel, M. Segal, E. Szanton, B. Weissbourd. 2003. *Caring for infants and toddlers in groups: Developmentally appropriate practice*. Arlington, VA: Zero to Three.
9. Endres, J. B., R. E. Rockwell. 2003. *Food, nutrition, and the young child*. 4th ed. New York: Macmillan.
10. Stang, J., C. T. Bayerl, M. M. Flatt. 2006. Position of the American Dietetic Association: Child and adolescent food and nutrition programs. *J American Dietetic Assoc* 106:1467-75.
11. Pipes, P. L., C. M. Trahms, eds. 1997. *Nutrition in infancy and childhood*. 6th ed. New York: McGraw-Hill.
12. William, C. O., ed. 1998. *Pediatric manual of clinical dietetics*. Chicago: American Dietetic Association.
13. Tamborlane, W. V., J. Warshaw, eds. 1997. *The Yale guide to children's nutrition*. New Haven, CT: Yale University Press.
14. Sullivan, S. A., L. L. Birch. 1990. Pass the sugar, pass the salt: Experience dictates preference. *Devel Psych* 26:546-51.
15. Murph, J. R., S. D. Palmer, D. Glassy, eds. 2005. *Health in child care: A manual for health professionals*. Elk Grove Village, IL: American Academy of Pediatrics.
16. Benjamin, S. E., D. F. Tate, S. I. Bangdiwala, B. H. Neelon, A. S. Ammerman, J. M. Dodds, D. S. Ward. 2008. Preparing child care health consultants to address childhood overweight: A randomized controlled trial comparing web to in-person training. *Maternal Child Health J* 12:662-69.
17. Ammerman, A. S., D. S. Ward, S. E. Benjamin, et al. 2007. An intervention to promote healthy weight: Nutrition and physical activity self-assessment for child care theory and design. *Public Health Research, Practice, and Policy* 4:1-12.
18. Story, M., K. M. Kaphingst, S. French. 2006. The role of child care settings in the prevention of obesity. *The Future of Children* 16:143-68
19. Dietz, W., L. Birch. 2008. *Eating behaviors of young child: Prenatal and postnatal influences on healthy eating*. Elk Grove Village, IL: American Academy of Pediatrics.

Health, Nutrition, Physical Activity, and Safety Awareness

STANDARD: Early care and education programs should have and implement written program plans addressing the health, nutrition, physical activity, and safety aspects of each formally structured activity documented in the written curriculum. These plans should include daily opportunities to learn health habits that prevent infection and significant injuries, and health habits that support healthful eating, nutrition education, and physical motor activity.

Awareness of healthy and safe behaviors, including good nutrition and physical activity, should be an integral part of the overall program.

RATIONALE: Young children learn better through experiencing an activity and observing behavior than through didactic methods (1). There may be a reciprocal relationship between learning and play so that play experiences are closely related to learning (2,3). Children can live by rules about health and safety when their personal experience helps them to understand why these rules were created. National guidelines for children birth to age five encourage their engagement in daily physical activity that promotes movement, motor skills and the foundations of health-related fitness (4). Physical activity is important to overall health and to overweight and obesity prevention (5).

COMMENTS: Resources for activities can be found at:

Fit Source - http://nccic.acf.hhs.gov/fitsource

Go Out and Play - http://www.cdc.gov/ncbddd/actearly/pdf/ccp_pdfs/GOP_kit.pdf

Center of Excellence for Training and Research Translation - www.center-trt.org

RELATED STANDARDS:

Socialization During Meals

Experience with Familiar and New Foods

Nutrition Learning Experiences for Children

Active Opportunities for Physical Activity

Appendix - Enjoy Moving: Be Physically Active Every Day

REFERENCES:

1. Fleer, M., ed. 1996. *Play through profiles: Profiles through play*. Watson, Australia: Australian Early Childhood Association.

2. Evaldson, A., W. A. Corsaro. 1998. Play and games in the peer cultures of preschool and preadolescent children: An interpretative approach. *Childhood* 5:377-402.

3. Petersen, E. A. 1998. The amazing benefits of play. *Child Family* 17:7-8.

4. National Association for Sport and Physical Education. 2009. *Active start: A statement of physical activity guidelines for children birth to five years*. 2nd ed. Reston, VA: NASPE.

5. U.S. Department of Health and Human Services, U.S. Department of Agriculture. 2005. *Dietary guidelines for Americans*. 6th ed. Washington, DC: U.S. Government Printing Office. http://www.health.gov/dietaryguidelines/dga2005/document/pdf/DGA2005.pdf.

Nutrition Education for Parents/Guardians

STANDARD: Parents/guardians should be informed of the range of nutrition learning activities provided in the facility. Formal nutrition information and education programs should be conducted at least twice a year under the guidance of the Nutritionist/Registered Dietitian based on a needs assessment for nutrition information and education as perceived by families and staff. Informal programs should be implemented during the "teachable moments" throughout the year.

RATIONALE: One goal of a facility is to provide a positive environment for the entire family. Informing parents/guardians about nutrition, food, food preparation, and mealtime enhances nutrition and mealtime interactions in the home, which helps to mold a child's food habits and eating behavior (1-9). Because of the current epidemic of childhood obesity, prevention of childhood obesity through nutrition and physical activity is an appropriate topic for parents/guardians. Periodically providing families records of the food eaten and progress in physical activities by their children will help families coordinate home food preparation, nutrition, and physical activity with what is provided at the early care and education facility. Nutrition education directed at parents/guardians complements and enhances the nutrition learning experiences provided to their children.

COMMENTS: One method of nutrition education for parents/guardians is providing healthy recipes that are quick and inexpensive to prepare and sharing information regarding access to local sources of healthy foods (farmers' markets, grocery stores, healthier prepared foods and restaurant options). Also caregivers/teachers can provide parents/guardians ideas for healthy and inexpensive snacks including foods available and served at parents' meetings. Education should be helpful, culturally relevant and incorporate the use of locally produced food. The educational programs may be supplemented by periodic distribution of newsletters and/or literature.

RELATED STANDARDS:
Nutrition Learning Experiences For Children (contains resources for nutrition expertise)

REFERENCES:
1. U.S. Department of Health and Human Services, Administration for Children and Families, Office of Head Start. 2009. *Head Start program performance standards*. Rev. ed. Washington, DC: U.S. Government Printing Office. http://eclkc.ohs.acf.hhs.gov/hslc/Program%20Design%20and%20 Management/Head%20Start%20Requirements/Head%20Start%20 Requirements/45%20CFR%20Chapter%20XIII/45%20CFR%20Chap%20 XIII_ENG.pdf.
2. Hagan, J. F., J. S. Shaw, P. M. Duncan, eds. 2008. *Bright futures: Guidelines for health supervision of infants, children, and adolescents*. 3rd ed. Elk Grove Village, IL: American Academy of Pediatrics.
3. Benjamin, S. E., ed. 2007. *Making food healthy and safe for children: How to meet the national health and safety performance standards – Guidelines for out of home child care programs*. 2nd ed. Chapel Hill, NC: National Training Institute for Child Care Health Consultants. http://nti.unc.edu/course_files/curriculum/nutrition/making_food_healthy_and_safe.pdf.
4. Dietz, W. H., L. Stern, eds. 1998. *American Academy of Pediatrics guide to your child's nutrition*. New York: Villard.
5. Endres, J. B., R. E. Rockwell. 2003. *Food, nutrition, and the young child*. 4th ed. New York: Macmillan.
6. U.S. Department of Agriculture. 2002. *Making nutrition count for children - Nutrition guidance for child care homes*. Washington, DC: USDA.
7. Pipes, P. L., C. M. Trahms, eds. 1997. *Nutrition in infancy and childhood*. 6th ed. New York: McGraw-Hill.
8. Tamborlane, W. V., ed. 1997. *The Yale guide to children's nutrition*. New Haven, CT: Yale University Press.
9. Kleinman, R. E., ed. 2009. *Pediatric nutrition handbook*. 6th ed. Elk Grove Village, IL: American Academy of Pediatrics.

Policies

Food and Nutrition Service Policies and Plans

STANDARD: The facility should have food handling, feeding, and nutrition policies and plans under the direction of the administration that address the following items and assign responsibility for each:

a) Kitchen layout;
b) Food budget;
c) Food procurement and storage;
d) Menu and meal planning;
e) Food preparation and service;
f) Kitchen and meal service staffing;
g) Nutrition education for children, staff, and parents/guardians;
h) Emergency preparedness for nutrition services;
i) Food brought from home including food brought for celebrations;
j) Age-appropriate portion sizes of food to meet nutritional needs;
k) Age-appropriate eating utensils and tableware;
l) Promotion of breastfeeding and provision of community resources to support mothers.

A Nutritionist/Registered Dietitian and a food service expert should provide input for and facilitate the development and implementation of a written nutrition plan for the early care and education facility.

RATIONALE: Having a plan that clearly assigns responsibility and that encompasses the pertinent nutrition elements will promote the optimal health of children and staff in early care and education settings.

For sample policies see the Nemours Health and Prevention Services guide on best practices for healthy eating at http://www.nemours.org/content/dam/nemours/www/filebox/service/preventive/nhps/heguide.pdf.

RELATED STANDARDS:
Written Nutrition Plan
Written Menu
General Plan for Feeding Infants
Feeding Infants on Cue by a Consistent Caregiver/Teacher
Preparing, Feeding, and Storing Human Milk
Serving Size for Toddlers and Preschoolers
Food Brought from Home
Use of Nutritionists/Registered Dietitians
Nutrition Learning Experiences for Children
Nutrition Education for Parents/Guardians
Appendix – Nutritionists/Registered Dietitians, Consultant, and Food Service Staff Qualifications
Appendix – Our Child Care Center Supports Breastfeeding

Infant Feeding Policy

STANDARD: A policy about infant feeding should be developed with the input and approval from the Nutritionist/Registered Dietitian and should include the following:

a) Storage and handling of expressed human milk;
b) Determination of the kind and amount of commercially prepared formula to be prepared for infants as appropriate;
c) Preparation, storage, and handling of infant formula;
d) Proper handwashing of the caregiver/teacher and the children;
e) Use and proper sanitizing of feeding chairs and of mechanical food preparation and feeding devices, including blenders, feeding bottles, and food warmers;

f) Whether expressed human milk, formula or infant food should be provided from home, and if so, how much food preparation and use of feeding devices, including blenders, feeding bottles, and food warmers, should be the responsibility of the caregiver/teacher;
g) Holding infants during bottle-feeding or feeding them sitting up;
h) Prohibiting bottle propping during feeding or prolonging feeding;
i) Responding to infants' need for food in a flexible fashion to allow cue feedings in a manner that is consistent with the developmental abilities of the child. Policy acknowledges that feeding infants on cue rather than on a schedule may help prevent obesity (1,2);
j) Introduction and feeding of age-appropriate solid foods (complementary foods);
k) Specification of the number of children who can be fed by one adult at one time;
l) Handling of food intolerance or allergies (examples include cow's milk, peanuts, orange juice, eggs, wheat).

Individual written infant feeding plans regarding feeding needs and feeding schedule should be developed for each infant in consultation with the infant's primary care provider and parents/guardians.

RATIONALE: Growth and development during infancy require that nourishing, wholesome, and developmentally appropriate food be provided, using safe approaches to feeding. Because individual needs must be accommodated and improper practices can have dire consequences for the child's health and safety, the policy for infant feeding should be developed with professional Nutritionists/Registered Dietitians. The infant feeding plans should be developed with each infant's parents/guardians and, when appropriate, in collaboration with the child's primary care provider.

RELATED STANDARDS:

General Plan for Feeding Infants
Feeding Infants on Cue by a Consistent Caregiver/Teacher
Preparing, Feeding, and Storing Human Milk
Feeding Human Milk to Another Mother's Child
Preparing, Feeding, and Storing Infant Formula
Techniques for Bottle Feeding
Introduction of Age-Appropriate Solid Foods to Infants
Feeding Age-Appropriate Solid Foods to Infants
Appendix - Our Child Care Center Supports Breastfeeding

REFERENCES:

1. Birch, L., W. Dietz. 2008. *Eating behaviors of young child: Prenatal and postnatal influences on healthy eating*, 59-93. Elk Grove Village, IL: American Academy of Pediatrics.
2. Taveras, E. M., S. L. Rifas-Shiman, K. S. Scanlon, L. M. Grummer-Strawn, B. Sherry, M. W. Gillman. 2006. To what extent is the protective effect of breastfeeding on future overweight explained by decreased maternal feeding restriction? *Pediatrics* 118:2341-48.

PHYSICAL ACTIVITY STANDARDS

Introduction

Physical activity and movement are an essential part of the development, learning, and growth of young children. During the first six years of life, infants, toddlers, and preschoolers are learning fundamental gross motor skills, and need ample opportunities to practice these skills. Recent evidence suggests that children may be more attentive and learn better after periods of activity and movement (1-4). Notably, physical activity is also a crucial part of maintaining a healthy weight and preventing obesity. Physical activity habits are established early in life and tracked over time (5-8). Therefore the preschool years are a key time in which to instill healthy physical activity habits that will last a lifetime, primarily through active play.

Although physical activity is essential to young children's growth and learning, there are potential barriers to daily opportunities for active play, including concerns about children's safety, time, curricular constraints, and inadequate knowledge or training among caregivers/teachers about how to integrate these opportunities into the curriculum. The following guidelines address common barriers to children's opportunities for activity and discuss ideas of how to incorporate physical activity safely and seamlessly into other programming activities.

REFERENCES:

1. Barros, R. M., E. J. Silver, R. E. Stein. 2009. School recess and group classroom behavior. *Pediatrics* 123:431-36.
2. Burdette, H. L., R. C. Whitaker. 2005. Resurrecting free play in young children: Looking beyond fitness and fatness to attention, affiliation, and affect. *Arch Pediatr Adolesc Med* 159:46-50.
3. Pellegrini, A., C. Bohn. 2005. The role of recess in children's cognitive performance and school adjustment. *Educ Res* 34:13-19.
4. Tomporowski, P. D., C. L. Davis, P. H. Miller, J. A. Naglieri. 2008. Exercise and children's intelligence, cognition, and academic achievement. *Educ Psychol Rev* 20:111-31.
5. Sallis, J. F., J. J. Prochaska, W. C. Taylor. 2000. A review of correlates of physical activity of children and adolescents. *Med Sci Sports Exerc* 32:963-75.
6. Sallis, J. F., C. C. Berry, S. L. Broyles, T. L. McKenzie, P. R. Nader. 1995. Variability and tracking of physical activity over 2 yr in young children. *Med Sci Sports Exerc* 27:1042-49.
7. McKenzie, T. L., J. F. Sallis, P. R. Nader, S. L. Broyles, J. A. Nelson. 1992. Anglo- and Mexican-American preschoolers at home and at recess: Activity patterns and environmental influences. *J Dev Behav Pediatr* 13:173-80.
8. Pate, R. R., T. Baranowski, M. Dowda, S. G. Trost. 1996. Tracking of physical activity in young children. *Med Sci Sports Exerc* 28:92-96.

Active Opportunities for Physical Activity

STANDARD: The facility should promote children's active play every day. Children should have ample opportunity to do vigorous activities such as running, climbing, dancing, skipping, and jumping. All children, birth to six years, should participate daily in:

a) Two to three occasions of active play outdoors, weather permitting (see Standard on Playing Outdoors for appropriate weather conditions);
b) Two or more structured or caregiver/teacher/adult-led activities or games that promote movement over the course of the day—indoor or outdoor;
c) Continuous opportunities to develop and practice age-appropriate gross motor and movement skills.

The total time allotted for outdoor play and vigorous indoor or outdoor physical activity can be adjusted for the age group and weather conditions.

a) Outdoor play:
  1) Infants (birth to twelve months of age) should be taken outside two to three times per day, as tolerated. There is no recommended duration of infants' outdoor play;
  2) Toddlers (twelve months to three years) and preschoolers (three to six years) should be allowed sixty to ninety total minutes of outdoor play. These outdoor times can be curtailed somewhat during adverse weather conditions in which children may still play safely outdoors for shorter periods, but should increase the time of indoor activity, so the total amount of exercise should remain the same;
b) Total time allotted for vigorous activities:
  1) Toddlers should be allowed sixty to ninety minutes per eight-hour day for vigorous physical activity, including running;

2) Preschoolers should be allowed ninety to one hundred and twenty minutes per eight-hour day (4).

Infants should have supervised tummy time every day when they are awake. Beginning on the first day at the early care and education program, caregivers/teachers should interact with an awake infant on their tummy for short periods of time (three to five minutes), increasing the amount of time as the infant shows he/she enjoys the activity (27).

Time spent outdoors has been found to be a strong, consistent predictor of children's physical activity (1-3). Children can accumulate opportunities for activity over the course of several shorter segments of at least ten minutes each. Because structured activities have been shown to produce higher levels of physical activity in young children, it is recommended that caregivers/teachers incorporate two or more short structured activities (five to ten minutes) or games daily that promote physical activity.

Opportunities to be actively enjoying physical activity should be incorporated into part-time programs by prorating these recommendations accordingly, i.e., twenty minutes of outdoor play for every three hours in the facility.

Active play should never be withheld from children who misbehave (e.g., child is kept indoors to help another caregiver/teacher while the rest of the children go outside) (5). However, children with out-of-control behavior may need five minutes or less to calm themselves or settle down before resuming cooperative play or activities.

Children should not be seated for more than fifteen minutes at a time, except during meals or naps. Infant equipment such as swings, stationary activity centers (ex. exersaucers), infant seats (ex. bouncers), molded seats, etc. if used should only be used for short periods of time. A least restrictive environment should be encouraged at all times. (5,6, 26).

Children should have adequate space for both inside and outside play.

RATIONALE: Free play, active play and outdoor play are essential components of young children's development (2). Children learn through play, developing gross motor, socio-emotional, and cognitive skills. In outdoor play, children learn about their environment, science, and nature.

Infants' and young children's participation in physical activity is critical to their overall health, development of motor skills, social skills, and maintenance of healthy weight (7). Daily physical activity promotes young children's gross motor development and provides numerous health benefits including improved fitness and cardiovascular health, healthy bone development, improved sleep, and improved mood and sense of well-being. Tummy time prepares infants for the time when they will be able to slide on their bellies and crawl. As infants grow older and stronger they will need more time on their tummies to build their own strength (27).

Daily physical activity is an important part of preventing excessive weight gain and childhood obesity. Some evidence also suggests that children may be able to learn better during or immediately after bursts of physical activity, due to improved attention and focus (8,9).

Numerous reports suggest that children are not meeting daily recommendations for physical activity, and that children spend 70% (10) to 87% (11) of their time in early care and education being sedentary, i.e., sitting or lying down. Excluding nap time, children are sedentary 83% of the time (11). Children may only spend about 2% to 3% of time being moderately or vigorously active (11).

Very young children are entirely dependent on their caregivers/teachers for opportunities to be active (12-15). Especially for children in full-time care and for children who live in unsafe neighborhoods, the early care and education facility may provide the child's only daily opportunity for active play. Evidence suggests that physical activity habits learned early in life may track into adolescence and adulthood supporting the importance for children to learn lifelong healthy physical activity habits while in the early care and education program (13,16-25).

COMMENTS: There are many ways to promote tummy time with infants:

1. Place yourself or a toy just out of the infant's reach during playtime to get him to reach for you or the toy;
2. Place toys in a circle around the infant. Reaching to different points in the circle will allow him/her to develop the appropriate muscles to roll over, scoot on his/her belly, and crawl;
3. Lie on your back and place the infant on your chest. The infant will lift his/her head and use his/her arms to try to see your face (27).

There are a multitude of short, structured activities that are appropriate for toddlers and preschoolers. Structured activities could include popular children's games such as Simon Says, Mother May I, Red Rover, Get the Wiggles Out, Musical Chairs, or a simple walk through the neighborhood. For training materials and more ideas of effective and age-appropriate games for young children, consider the following resources:

- Nutrition and Physical Activity Self Assessment for

Child Care - NAP SACC Program - http://www.napsacc.org;
- "Color Me Healthy Preschoolers Moving and Eating"- http://www.colormehealthy.com
- "Move and Learn" physical activity curriculum from Kansas State University;
- "I am Moving I am Learning" Intervention in Head Start - http://eclkc.ohs.acf.hhs.gov/hslc/ecdh/Health/Nutrition/Nutrition%20Program%20Staff/IamMovinglam.htm;
- Moving and Learning: The Physical Activity Specialists for Birth through Age 8 - http://www.movingandlearning.com;
- "How to Lower Your Risk for Type 2 Diabetes "National Diabetes Education Program http://ndep.nih.gov/media/kids-tips-lower-risk.pdf.

Experts disagree about the appropriate amount of physical activity for toddlers and preschoolers, what proportion of children's physical activity should be structured, and to what extent structured activities are effective in producing children's physical activity. Researchers do agree that toddlers and preschoolers generally accumulate vigorous physical activity over the course of the day in very short bursts (fifteen to thirty seconds) (23). For additional recommendations by other national groups and experts, see:

a) The National Association for Sport and Physical Education's *Active Start: A Statement of Physical Activity Guidelines for Children From Birth to Age 5, 2nd Edition* at http://www.aahperd.org/naspe/standards/nationalGuidelines/ActiveStart.cfm and *Physical Activity for Children: A Statement of Guidelines for Children 5 - 12, 2nd Edition* at http://www.aahperd.org/naspe/standards/nationalGuidelines/PA-Children-5-12.cfm;

b) U.S. Department of Health and Human Services' *2008 Physical Activity Guidelines for Americans* at http://www.health.gov/PAGuidelines/Report/pdf/CommitteeReport.pdf ;

c) U.S. Department of Health and Human Services and the U.S. Department of Agriculture's *Dietary Guidelines for Americans, 2005* at http://www.health.gov/dietaryguidelines/dga2005/document/default.htm.

RELATED STANDARDS:

Health, Nutrition, Physical Activity, and Safety Awareness
Caregivers/Teachers' Encouragement of Physical Activity
Policies and Practices that Promote Physical Activity
Appendix – Enjoy Moving: Be Physically Active Every Day

REFERENCES:

1. Brown, W. H., K. A. Pfeiffer, K. L. McIver, M. Dowda, C. L. Addy, R. R. Pate. 2009. Social and environmental factors associated with preschoolers' nonsedentary physical activity. *Child Development* 80:45-58.
2. Burdette, H. L., R. C. Whitaker. 2005. Resurrecting free play in young children: Looking beyond fitness and fatness to attention, affiliation, and affect. *Arch Pediatr Adolesc Med* 159:46-50.
3. Burdette, H. L., R. C. Whitaker, S. R. Daniels. 2004. Parental report of outdoor playtime as a measure of physical activity in preschool-aged children. *Arch Pediatr Adolesc Med* 158:353-57.
4. Bower, J. K., D. P. Hales, D. F. Tate, D. A. Rubin, S. E. Benjamin, D. S. Ward. 2008. The childcare environment and children's physical activity. *Am J Prev Med* 34:23-29.
5. Benjamin, S. E., A. Ammerman, J. Sommers, J. Dodds, B. Neelon, D. S. Ward. 2007. *The nutrition and physical activity self-assessment for child care (NAP SACC).* Rev ed. Raleigh and Chapel Hill, NC: UNC Center for Health Promotion and Disease Prevention, Center of Excellence for Training and Research Translation. http://www.center-trt.org/downloads/obesity_prevention/interventions/napsacc/NAPSACC_Template.pdf.
6. National Association for Sport and Physical Education. 2002. *Active start: A statement of physical activity guidelines for children birth to five years.* Washington, DC: NASPE.
7. Patrick, K., B. Spear, K. Holt, D. Sofka, eds. 2001. *Bright futures in practice: Physical activity.* Arlington, VA: National Center for Education in Maternal and Child Health. http://www.brightfutures.org/physicalactivity/pdf/index.html.
8. Pellegrini, A., C. Bohn. 2005. The role of recess in children's cognitive performance and school adjustment. *Educ Res* 34:13-19.
9. Mahar, M. T., S. K. Murphy, D. A. Rowe, J. Golden, A. T. Shields, T. D. Raedeke. 2006. Effects of a classroom-based program on physical activity and on-task behavior. *Med Sci Sports Exerc* 38:2086-94.
10. Pate, R. R., K. A. Pfeiffer, S. G. Trost, P. Ziegler, M. Dowda. 2004. Physical activity among children attending preschools. *Pediatrics* 114:1258-63.
11. Pate, R. R., K. McIver, M. Dowda, W. H. Brown, A. Cheryl. 2008. Directly observed physical activity levels in preschool children. *J Sch Health* 78:438-44.
12. McKenzie, T. L., J. F. Sallis, J. P. Elder, C. C. Berry, P. L. Hoy, P. R. Nader, M. M. Zive, S. L. Broyles. 1997. Physical activity levels and prompts in young children at recess: A two-year study of a bi-ethnic sample. *Res Q Exerc Sport* 68:195-202.
13. McKenzie, T. L., J. F. Sallis, P. R. Nader, S. L. Broyles, J. A. Nelson. 1992. Anglo- and Mexican-American preschoolers at home and at recess: Activity patterns and environmental influences. *J Dev Behav Pediatr* 13:173-80.
14. Sallis, J. F., T. L. McKenzie, J. P. Elder, S. L. Broyles, P. R. Nader. 1997. Factors parents use in selecting play spaces for young children. *Arch Pediatr Adolesc Med* 151:414-17.
15. Sallis, J. F., P. R. Nader, S. L. Broyles, J. P. Elder, T. L. McKenzie, J. A. Nelson. 1993. Correlates of physical activity at home in Mexican-American and Anglo-American preschool children. *Health Psychol* 12:390-98.
16. Davis, K., K. K. Christoffel. 1994. Obesity in preschool and school-age children: Treatment early and often may be best. *Arch Pediatr Adolesc Med* 148:1257-61.
17. Sallis, J. F., C. C. Berry, S. L. Broyles, T. L. McKenzie, P. R. Nader. 1995. Variability and tracking of physical activity over 2 yr in young children. *Med Sci Sports Exerc* 27:1042-49.
18. Pate, R. R., T. Baranowski, S. G. Trost. 1996. Tracking of physical activity in young children. *Med Sci Sports Exerc* 28:92-96.
19. Birch, L. L., J. O. Fisher. 1998. Development of eating behaviors among children and adolescents. *Pediatrics* 101:539-49.

20. Sallis, J. F., J. J. Prochaska, W. C. Taylor. 2000. A review of correlates of physical activity of children and adolescents. *Med Sci Sports Exerc* 32:963-75.
21. Skinner, J. D., B. R. Carruth, W. Bounds, P. Ziegler, K. Reidy. 2002. Do food-related experiences in the first 2 years of life predict dietary variety in school-aged children? *J Nutr Educ Behav* 34:310-15.
22. Skinner, J. D., B. R. Carruth, B. Wendy, P. J. Ziegler. 2002. Children's food: A longitudinal analysis. *J Am Diet Assoc* 102:1638-47.
23. Oliver, M., G. M. Schofield, G. S. Kolt. 2007. Physical activity in pre-schoolers: Understanding prevalence and measurement issues. *Sports Med* 37:1045-70.
24. American Academy of Pediatrics, Council on Sports Medicine and Fitness, and Council on School Health. 2006. Active healthy living: Prevention of childhood obesity through increased physical activity. *Pediatrics* 117:1834-42.
25. Physical Activity Guidelines Advisory Committee. 2008. *Physical activity guidelines advisory committee report, 2008.* Washington, D.C.: U.S. Department of Health and Human Services. http://www.health.gov/PAGuidelines/Report/pdf/CommitteeReport.pdf.
26. American Physical Therapy Association. 2008. *Lack of time on tummy shown to hinder achievement of developmental milestones, say physical therapists.* http://www.apta.org/AM/Template.cfm?Section=Home&Template=/CM/ContentDisplay.cfm&ContentID=57947.
27. American Academy of Pediatrics. 2008. Back to sleep, tummy to play. Elk Grove Village, IL: American Academy of Pediatrics. http://www.healthychildcare.org/pdf/SIDStummytime.pdf.

Playing Outdoors

STANDARD: Children should play outdoors daily when weather and environmental conditions do not pose a significant health or safety risk. Outdoor play for infants may include riding in a carriage or stroller; however, infants should be offered opportunities for gross motor play outdoors, as well.

Weather that poses a significant health risk should include wind chill factor at or below minus 15°F and heat index at or above 90°F, as identified by the National Weather Service.

Children should be protected from the sun by using shade, sun-protective clothing, and sunscreen with UVB-ray and UVA-ray protection of SPF 15 or higher, with permission from parents/guardians. Before prolonged physical activity in warm weather, children should be well-hydrated and should be encouraged to drink water during the activity. On hot days, infants receiving human milk in a bottle can be given additional human milk in a bottle but should not be given water, especially in the first six months of life. Infants receiving formula and water can be given additional formula in a bottle. In warm weather, children's clothing should be light-colored, lightweight, and limited to one layer of absorbent material to facilitate the evaporation of sweat. Children should wear sun-protective clothing, such as hats, when playing outdoors between the hours of 10 AM and 2 PM.

In cold weather, children's clothing should be layered and dry. Caregivers/teachers should check children's extremities for maintenance of normal color and warmth at least every fifteen minutes when children are outdoors in cold weather. When precipitation is present (such as rain or snow), children should be properly clothed (boots, gloves, hats, etc.) to participate in outdoor play.

Caregivers/teachers should also be aware of environmental hazards such as contaminated water, loud noises, and lead in soil when selecting an area to play outdoors. Children should be observed closely when playing in dirt/soil, so that no soil is ingested. Play areas should be secure and away from heavy traffic areas.

RATIONALE: Outdoor play is not only an opportunity for learning in a different environment; it also provides many health benefits. Outdoor play allows for physical activity that supports maintenance of a healthy weight (2). Light exposure of the skin to sunlight promotes the production of vitamin D that growing children require.

Open spaces in outdoor areas, even those confined to screened rooftops in urban play spaces, encourage children to develop gross motor skills and fine motor play in ways that are difficult to duplicate indoors. Nevertheless, some weather conditions make outdoor play hazardous.

Caregivers/teachers must protect children from adverse weather and air quality. Wind chill conditions that pose a risk of frostbite as well as heat and humidity that pose a significant risk of heat-related illness are defined by the National Weather Service and are announced routinely. The federal government has established health standards for a number of air pollutants. Caregivers/teachers should consult this information.

Heat-induced illness and cold injury are preventable. Children have greater surface area-to-body mass ratio than adults. Therefore, children do not adapt to extremes of temperature as effectively as adults when exposed to a high climatic heat stress or to cold. Children produce more metabolic heat per mass unit than adults when walking or running. They also have a lower sweating capacity and cannot dissipate body heat by evaporation as effectively (1).

Generally, infectious disease organisms are less concentrated in outdoor air than indoor air.

COMMENTS: The National Weather Service provides convenient color-coded guides for caregivers/teachers to

use to determine which weather conditions are comfortable for outdoor play, which require caution, and which are dangerous. These guides are available on the National Weather Service Website at http://www.nws.noaa.gov/om/windchill/index.shtml for wind chill and http://www.nws.noaa.gov/om/heat/index.shtml for heat index. The federal Clean Air Act requires that the Environmental Protection Agency (EPA) establish ambient air quality health standards. Most local health departments monitor weather and air quality in their jurisdiction and make appropriate announcements.

To access the latest local weather information and warnings, contact the National Weather Service at http://www.weather.gov/.

Winter can be problematic for children with asthma for two reasons. Indoor allergens such as dust and dust mites are common triggers for asthma symptoms and levels of these allergens can become elevated during the winter, when doors and windows are kept shut to keep out cold air. Cold temperatures also may, in some cases, serve as a trigger to asthma symptoms for children with asthma. Children for whom cold weather is an asthma trigger may be helped by wearing a scarf during periods of cold weather. All children with asthma can safely play outdoors as long as their asthma is well controlled, and the parents/guardians of children with asthma should be encouraged to work with their child's primary care provider to develop a plan the child can self-manage that incorporates opportunities for outdoor play.

The thought is often expressed that children are more likely to become sick if exposed to cold air, however upper respiratory infections and flu are caused by viruses, not exposure to cold air. These viruses spread easily during the winter when children are kept indoors in close proximity. The best protection against the spread of illness is regular and proper handwashing for both children and caregivers/teachers, as well as proper sanitation procedures during mealtimes, and when there is any contact with bodily fluids.

RELATED STANDARDS:

Active Opportunities for Physical Activity
Caregivers/Teachers' Encouragement of Physical Activity
Appendix – Enjoy Moving: Be Physically Active Every Day

REFERENCES:

1. American Academy of Pediatrics, Committee on Sports Medicine and Fitness. 2000. Climatic heat stress and the exercising child and adolescent. *Pediatrics* 106:158-59.

2. Hagan, J. F., J. S. Shaw, P. M. Duncan, eds. 2008. Promoting physical activity. In *Bright futures: Guidelines for health supervision of infants, children, and adolescents*, 147-54. 3rd ed. Elk Grove Village, IL: American Academy of Pediatrics.

Caregivers/Teachers' Encouragement of Physical Activity

STANDARD: Caregivers/teachers should promote children's active play, and participate in children's active games at times when they can safely do so. Caregivers/teachers should:

a) Lead structured activities to promote children's activities two or more times per day;
b) Wear clothing and footwear that permits easy and safe movement;
c) Not sit during active play;
d) Provide prompts for children to be active, e.g., "good throw";
e) Encourage children's physical activities that are appropriate and safe in the setting , e.g. do not prohibit running on the playground when it is safe to run;
f) Have orientation and annual training opportunities to learn about age-appropriate gross motor activities and games that promote children's physical activity;
g) Limit screen time (TV, DVD, computer).

RATIONALE: Children learn from the modeling of healthy and safe behavior.

Chairs for adults on playgrounds inhibit the promotion of children's physical activity. They may also pose a safety hazard if caregivers/teachers sitting in them cannot see all parts of the playground.

COMMENTS: Caregivers/teachers may not feel comfortable promoting active play, perhaps due to inhibitions about their own physical activity skills, or due to lack of training. Caregivers/teachers may feel that their sole role on the playground is to supervise and keep children safe, rather than to promote physical activity. Continuing education activities are useful in disseminating knowledge about effective games to promote physical activity in early care and education while keeping children safe. Caregivers/teachers should consider incorporating structured activities into the curriculum indoors, or after children have been on playground for ten to fifteen minutes, as children tend to be less active after the first ten to fifteen minutes on the playground. Caregivers/teachers, if they are facilitating physical activity with a small group, must ensure that there is adequate supervision of all children on the playground.

Caregivers/teachers should be aware that there is often a high level of TV and computer exposure in the home. Early care and education settings offer caregivers/teachers the opportunity to model the limitation of media and computer time and to educate parents/guardians about alternative activities that families can do with their children.

RELATED STANDARDS:
Active Opportunities for Physical Activity
Playing Outdoors
Policies and Practices that Promote Physical Activity
Limiting Screen Time - Media, Computer, etc.
Appendix – Enjoy Moving: Being Physically Active Every Day

Policies and Practices that Promote Physical Activity

STANDARD: The facility should have written policies on the promotion of physical activity and the removal of potential barriers to physical activity participation. Policies should cover the following:

a) Benefits: benefits of physical activity and outdoor play;
b) Duration: children will spend sixty to ninety minutes each day outdoors depending on their age, weather permitting. Policies will describe what will be done to ensure physical activity on days with more extreme temperatures (either very hot or very cold);
c) Setting: provision of covered areas for shade and shelter on playgrounds, if feasible (2);
d) Clothing: clothing should permit easy movement (not too loose and not too tight) that enables children to participate fully in active play. Footwear should provide support for running and climbing:
   Examples of appropriate clothing/footwear include:
   1) Gym shoes or sturdy gym-shoe-equivalent;
   2) Clothes for the weather, including heavy coat, hat, and mittens in the winter/snow; raincoat and/or boots for the rain; and layered clothes for climates in which the temperature can vary dramatically on a daily basis;
   Examples of inappropriate clothing/footwear include:
   1) Footwear that can come off while running, or that provide insufficient support for climbing (3);
   2) Clothing that can catch on playground equipment (e.g. with drawstrings or loops).

If children wear "dress clothes" or special outfits that cannot be easily laundered, caregivers/teachers should talk with the children's parents/guardians about the program's goals in providing physical activity during the program day and encourage them to provide a set of clothes that can be used during physical activities.

Facilities should discuss the importance of this policy with parents/guardians upon enrollment and periodically thereafter.

In addition to outdoor play, the facility is encouraged to incorporate brief movement activities or games into the standard indoor curriculum.

RATIONALE: If appropriately dressed, children can safely play outdoors in most weather conditions. Children can learn math, science, and language concepts through games involving movement (1).

COMMENTS: Lack of coat, mittens/gloves, and/or hat has been cited as a barrier to children's physical activity in early care and education (3). Caregivers/teachers can mitigate this issue by having extra clean clothing on hand. Only when weather-related health alerts are issued should restrictions be placed on outdoor activity. Children can play in the rain, snow, and in low temperatures, when wearing clothing that keeps them dry and warm. When it is very warm, children can play outdoors, if they play in shady areas, wear sun-protective clothing, and have water available to mist or sprinkle and plenty of water available for drinking.

Having a policy on outdoor physical activity that will take place on days when weather is moderately (but not severely) inclement informs all caregivers/teachers and families about the facility's expectations. The policy can make clear that outdoor activity may require special clothing, in colder weather, or arrangements for cooling off, when it is warm. By having such a policy, the facility encourages caregivers/teachers and families to anticipate and prepare for outdoor activity when cold, hot, or wet weather prevails. The policy also identifies when alternate large muscle activity should be held indoors so that weather conditions do not dictate lack of physical activity.

For examples of policies, see the Nemours Health and Prevention Services guide on best practices for physical activity at: http://www.nemours.org/content/dam/nemours/www/filebox/service/preventive/nhps/heguide.pdf.

RELATED STANDARDS:

Active Opportunities to Promote Physical Activity
Playing Outdoors
Caregivers/Teachers' Encouragement of Physical Activity
Appendix – Enjoy Moving: Be Physically Active Every Day

REFERENCES:

1. Trost, S. G., B. Fees, D. Dzewaltowski. 2008. Feasibility and efficacy of a "move and learn" physical activity curriculum in preschool children. *J Phys Act Health* 5:88-103.

2. McWilliams, C., S. G. Ball, S. E. Benjamin, D. Hales, A. Vaughn, D. S. Ward. 2009. Best-practice guidelines for physical activity at child care. *Pediatrics* 124:1650-59.

3. Copeland, K. A., S. N. Sherman, C. A. Kendeigh, B. E. Saelens, H. J. Kalkwarf. 2009. Flip flops, dress clothes, and no coat: Clothing barriers to children's physical activity in child-care centers identified from a qualitative study. *Int J Behav Nutr and Physical Activity* 6, no. 74 (November 6). http://ijbnpa.org/content/6/1/74.

SCREEN TIME STANDARD

Limiting Screen Time – Media, Computer Time

STANDARD: In early care and education settings, media (television [TV], video, and DVD) viewing and computer use should not be permitted for children younger than two years. For children two years and older in early care and early education settings, total media time should be limited to not more than thirty minutes once a week, and for educational or physical activity use only. During meal or snack time, TV, video, or DVD viewing should not be allowed (1). Computer use should be limited to no more than fifteen-minute increments except for school-age children completing homework assignments (2).

Parents/guardians should be informed if screen media are used in the early care and education program. Any screen media used should be free of advertising and brand placement. TV programs, DVD, and computer games should be reviewed and evaluated before participation of the children to ensure that advertising and brand placement are not present.

RATIONALE: In the first two years of life, children's brains and bodies are going through critical periods of growth and development. It is important for infants and young children to have positive interactions with people and not sit in front of a screen that takes time away from social interaction with parents/guardians and caregivers/teachers. Before age three, television viewing can have modest negative effects on cognitive development of children (3). For that reason, the American Academy of Pediatrics (AAP) recommends television viewing be discouraged for children younger than two years of age (4). Interactive activities that promote brain development can be encouraged, such as talking, playing, singing, and reading together.

For children two years and older, the AAP recommends limiting children's total (early care and education, and home) media time (with entertainment media) to no more than one to two hours of quality programming per twenty-four hour period (3). Because children may watch television before and after attending early care and education settings, limiting media time during their time in early care and education settings will help meet the AAP recommendation. When TV watching is intended to be interactive, with the adult interacting with children about what they are watching, caregivers/teachers can sing along and comment on what children are watching. Caregivers/teachers should always consider whether children could learn the skill better in another way through hands-on experiences.

Studies have shown a relationship between TV viewing and overweight in young children. For example, watching more than eight hours of television per week has been associated with an increased risk of obesity in young children and exposure to two or more hours of television per day increased the risk of overweight for three-to five-year-olds (5,6). Among four-year-olds, as body mass index increased, average hours of TV viewing increased (7). Also, young children who watch TV have been shown to have poor diet quality. For each one-hour increment of TV viewing per day, three-year-olds were found to have higher intakes of sugar-sweetened beverage and lower fruit and vegetable intakes (8). Children are exposed to extensive advertising for high-calorie and low-nutrient dense foods and drinks and very limited advertising of healthful foods and drinks during their television viewing. Television advertising influences the food consumption of children two- to eleven-years-old (9).

About two-thirds (66%) of children ages six months to six years watch television every day. About a quarter (24%) watch videos or DVDs every day, and nearly two-thirds (65%) watch them several times a week or more. Additionally, young children engage in other forms of screen activity several times a week or more including using a computer (27%), playing console video games (13%) and playing handheld video games (8%) (10). Survey data show that by three months of age, about 40% of infants regularly watch television, DVDs or videos. By twenty-four months, this rose to 90% (1).

Caregivers/teachers cannot determine which child does and does not watch TV at home. It is important for early care and education programs to limit TV viewing so that the AAP goal of less than two hours a day, accompanied by more physical activity and increased interaction with reading, can be achieved. A study of TV viewing in early care and education settings reported that, on average, preschool-aged children watched more than four times as much television while at home-based programs than at center-based programs (1.39 hours per day vs. 0.36 hours per day); with significant differences between groups in the type of television content viewed, and in the proportions of programs in which no television viewing occurred at all. The proportion of programs where preschool-aged children watched no television during the early care and education day was 65% in center-based programs and 11% in home-based programs (11).

COMMENT: It is important for caregivers/teachers to be a role model for children in early care and education settings by not watching TV during the care day. In addition, when adults watch television (including the news) in the presence of children, children may be exposed to inappropriate language or frightening images. MyPyramid has tips on limiting media time - "How Much Inactive Time Is Too Much" at http://www.mypyramid.gov/preschoolers/PhysicalActivity/inactivetime.html.

The AAP provides a description of the TV programming rating scale and tips for parents/guardians at http://www.aap.org/publiced/BR_TV.htm. Caregivers/teachers are discouraged from having a TV in a room where children are present.

Caregivers/teachers should begin reading to children when they are six months of age and facilities should have age-appropriate books available for each cognitive stage of development. See "Reach Out and Read" at http://www.reachoutandread.org for more information.

RELATED STANDARDS:

Active Opportunities for Physical Activity

Appendix – Enjoy Moving: Be Physically Active Every Day

REFERENCES:

1. Zimmerman, F. J., D. A. Christakis, A. N. Meltzoff. 2007. Television and DVD/video viewing in children younger than 2 years. *Arch Pediatric Adolescent Med* 161:473-79.

2. Harms, T., R. M. Clifford, D. Cryer. 2005. Early childhood environment rating scale, revised ed. Frank Porter Graham Child Development Institute, University of North Carolina. http://www.fpg.unc.edu/~ECERS/.

3. Zimmerman, F. J., D. A. Christakis. 2005. Children's television viewing and cognitive outcomes. *Arch Pediatric Adolescent Med* 159:619-25.

4. American Academy of Pediatrics, Council on Communications and Media. 2009. Policy statement: Media violence. *Pediatrics* 124:1495-1503.

5. Reilly, J. J., J. Armstrong, A. R. Dorosty. 2005. Early life risk factors for obesity in childhood: Cohort study. *British Medical J* 330:1357.

6. Lumeng, J. C., S. Rahnama, D. Appugliese, N. Kaciroti, R. H. Bradley. 2006. Television exposure and overweight risk in preschoolers. *Arch Pediatric Adolescent Med* 160:417-22.

7. Levin, S., M. W. Martin, W. F. Riner. 2004. TV viewing habits and Body Mass Index among South Carolina Head Start children. *Ethnicity and Disease* 14:336-39.

8. Miller, S. A., E. M. Taveras, S. L. Rifas-Shiman, M. W. Gillman. 2008. Association between television viewing and poor diet quality in young children. *Int J Pediatric Obesity* 3:168-76.

9. Committee on Food Marketing and the Diets of Children and Youth. 2006. *Food marketing to children and youth: Threat or opportunity*. Eds. J. M. McGinnis, J. A. Gootman, V. I. Kraak. Washington, DC: National Academies Press.

10. Taveras, E. M., T. J. Sandora, M. C. Shih, D. Ross-Degnan, D. A. Goldmann, M. W. Gillman. 2006. The association of television and video viewing with fast food intake by preschool-age children. *Obesity* 14:2034-41.

11. Christakis, D. A., M. M. Garrison, F. J. Zimmerman. 2006. Television viewing in child care programs: A national survey. *Communication Reports* 19:111-20.

Additional Readings:

Dennison, B. A., T. A. Erb, P. L. Jenkins. 2002. Television viewing and television in bedroom associated with overweight risk among low-income preschool children. *Pediatrics* 109:1028-35.

Funk, J. B., J. Brouwer, K. Curtiss, E. McBroom. 2009. Parents of preschoolers: Expert media recommendations and ratings knowledge, media-effects beliefs, and monitoring practices. *Pediatrics* 123:981-88.

National Association for the Education of Young Children. 1994. Media violence in children's lives. Position Statement. http://www.naeyc.org/files/naeyc/file/positions/PSMEVI98.PDF.

Martinez-Gomez, D., J. Tucker, K. A. Heelan, G. J. Welk, J. C. Eisenmann. 2009. Associations between sedentary behavior and blood pressure in young children. *Arch Pediatr Adolesc Med* 163:724-30.

Nixon, G. M., J. M. D. Thompson, D. Y. Han, et al. 2009. Falling asleep: The determinants of sleep latency. *Arch Dis Child* 94:686-89.

McMurray, R. G., S. I. Bangdiwala, J. S. Harrell, L. D. Amorim. 2008. Adolescents with metabolic syndrome have a history of low aerobic fitness and physical activity levels. *Dynamic Med* 7:5.

McDonough, P. 2009. TV viewing among kids at an eight-year high. Nielsen Wire (October 26). http://blog.nielsen.com/nielsenwire/media_entertainment/tv-viewing-among-kids-at-an-eight-year-high/.

APPENDICES

MyPyramid for Preschoolers Mini-Poster

MyPyramid
for Preschoolers
Eat Right. Exercise. Have Fun.
MyPyramid.gov
GREEN BEANS
MILK
PEANUT BUTTER
TUNA
Grains
Make half your grains whole
Vegetables
Vary your veggies
Fruits
Focus on fruits
Milk
Get your calcium-rich foods
Meat & Beans
Go lean with protein
Oils
Oils are not a food group, but you need some for good health. Get your oils from fish, nuts, and liquid oils such as corn oil, soybean oil, and canola oil.
Find your balance between food and fun
Fats and sugars – know your limits
MyPyramid.gov
USDA
U.S. Department of Agriculture
September 2008
FNS-408
USDA is an equal opportunity provider and employer.

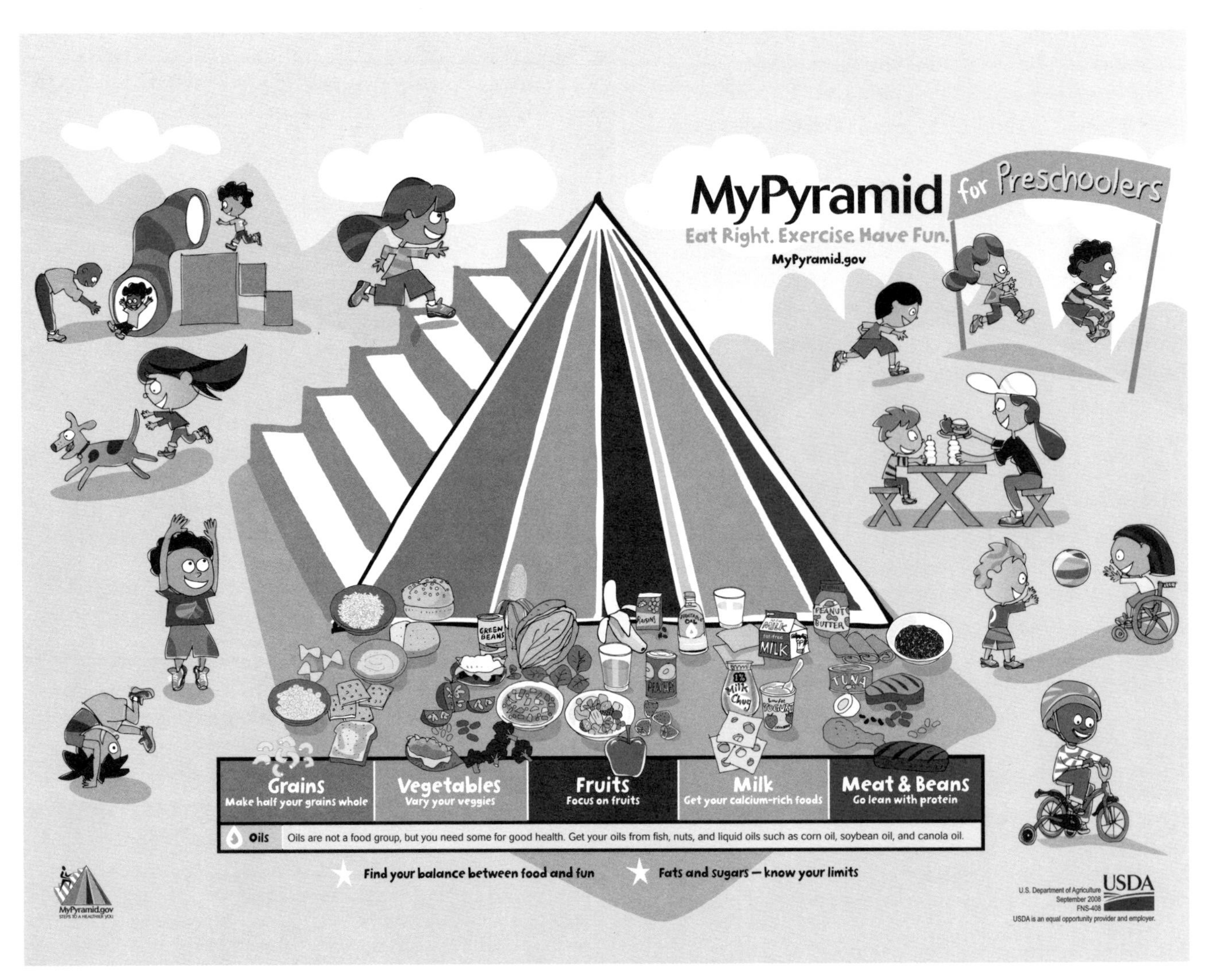

Note to Reader - This poster was current as of the print date for *Preventing Childhood Obesity in Early Care and Education Programs: Selected Standards from Caring for Our Children, 3rd Ed*. However, this poster is updated periodically - please check the current poster at http://www.mypyramid.gov/

Reference:
1. U.S. Department of Agriculture. 2008. MyPyramid for preschoolers. Arlington, VA: USDA. http://www.mypyramid.gov/downloads/PreschoolerMiniPoster.pdf.

MyPyramid for Kids Mini-Poster

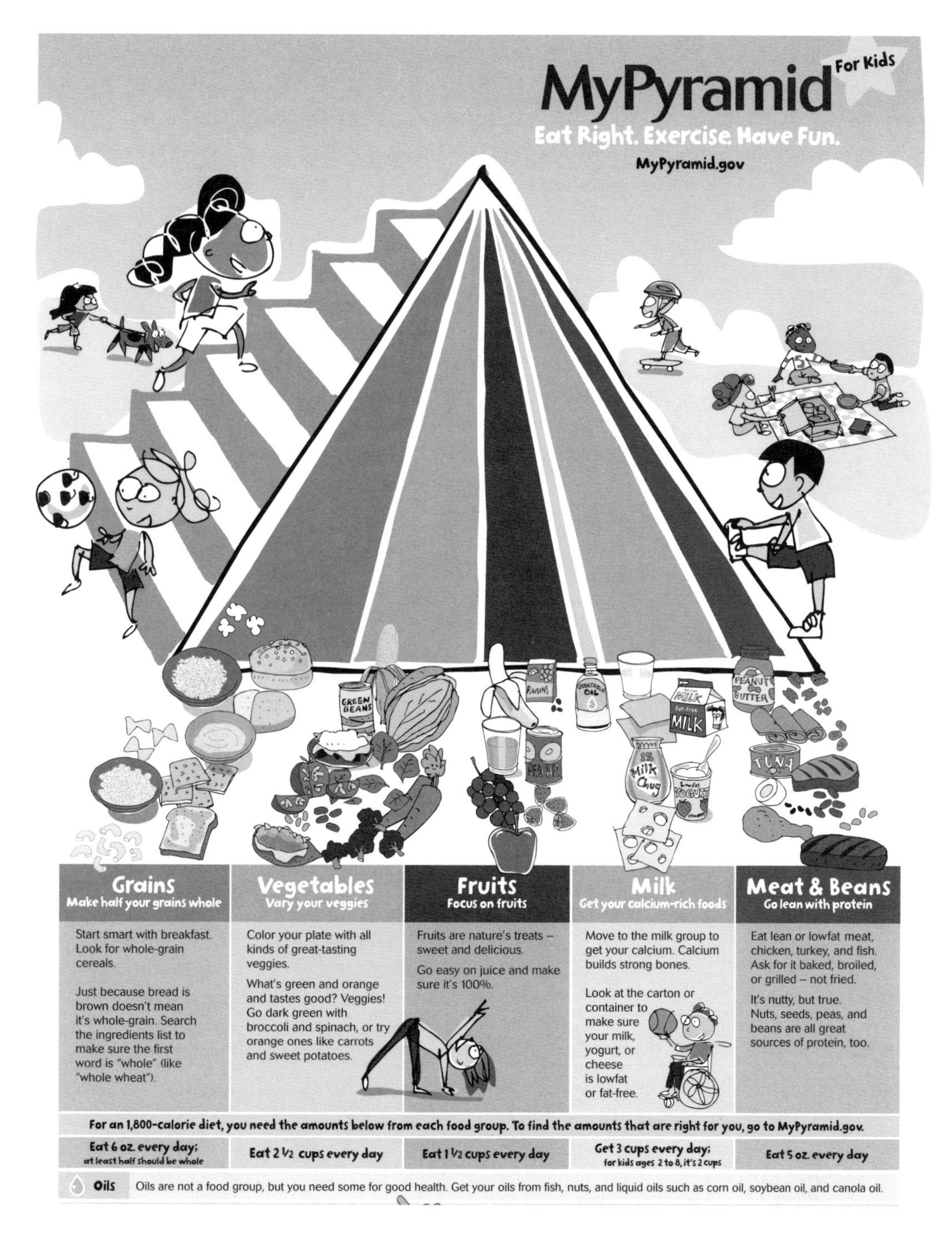

Note to Reader - This poster was current as of the print date for *Preventing Childhood Obesity in Early Care and Education Programs: Selected Standards from Caring for Our Children, 3rd Ed.* However, this poster is updated periodically - please check the current poster at http://www.mypyramid.gov/

Enjoy Moving: Be Physically Active Every Day

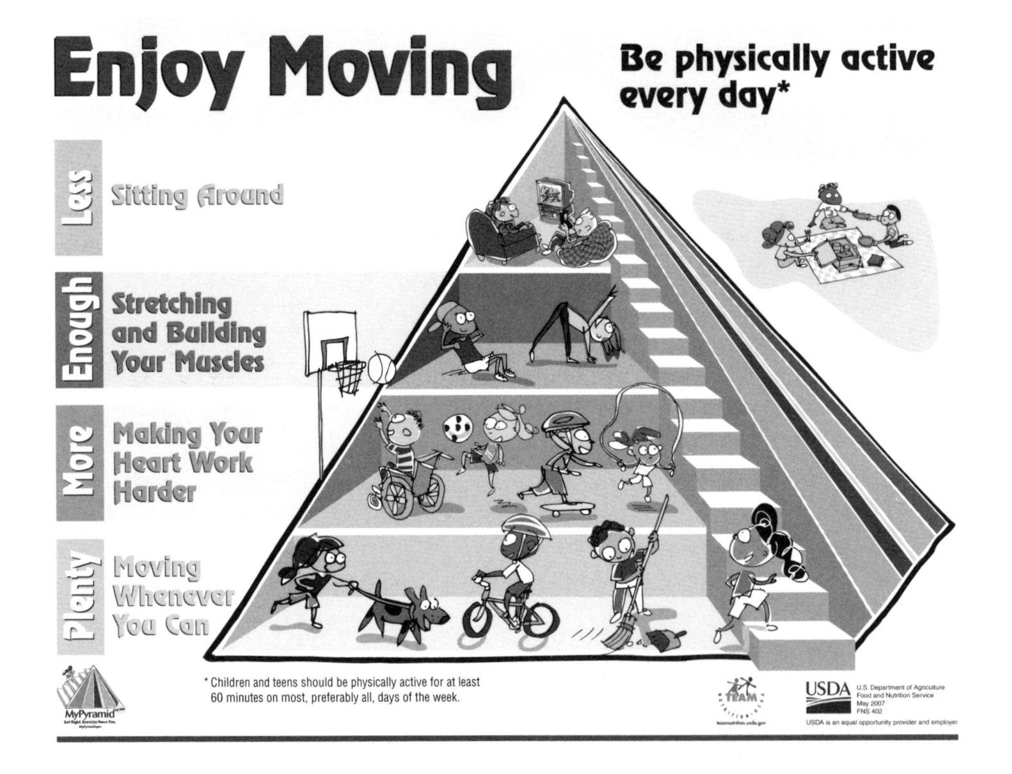

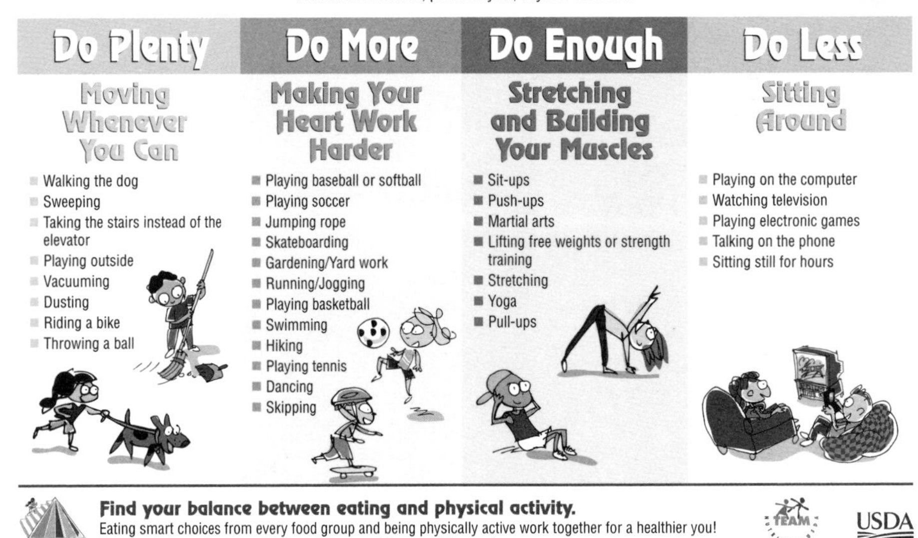

Note to Reader - This poster was current as of the print date for *Preventing Childhood Obesity in Early Care and Education Programs: Selected Standards from Caring for Our Children, 3rd Ed.* However, this poster is updated periodically - please check the current poster at http://www.mypyramid.gov/

Our Child Care Center Supports Breastfeeding

Because we are committed to healthy mothers and children,

Our Child Care Center Supports Breastfeeding

In order to support families who are breastfeeding or who are considering breastfeeding, we strive to do the following:

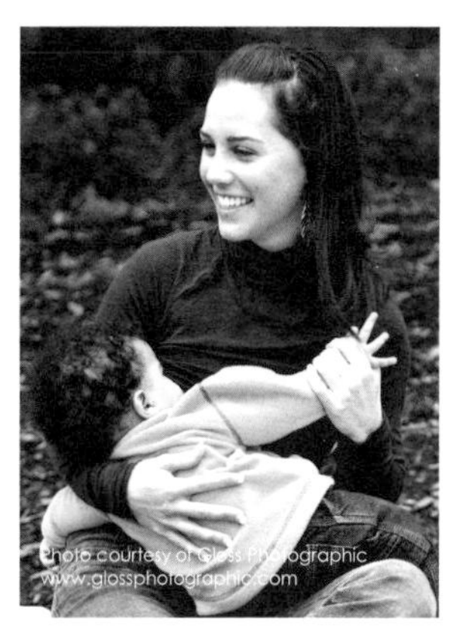

- Make a commitment to the importance of breastfeeding, especially exclusive breastfeeding, and proudly share this commitment with our staff and clients.
- Train all staff in supporting the best infant and young child feeding.
- Inform families about the importance of breastfeeding.
- Develop a breastfeeding-friendly feeding plan with each family.
- Train all staff to handle, store, and feed mother's milk properly.
- Teach our clients to properly store and label their milk for child care center use.

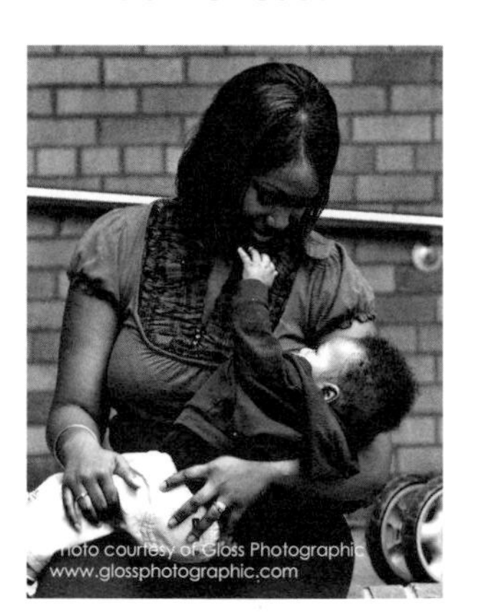

- Provide a breastfeeding-friendly environment, welcoming mothers to nurse their babies at our center.
- Display posters and brochures that support breastfeeding and show best practices.
- Contact and coordinate with local skilled breastfeeding support and actively refer.
- Continually update our information and learning about breastfeeding support.

Breastfeeding Families Welcome Here!

Breastfeeding-Friendly Child Care Initiative

A collaboration between Wake County's Child Care Health Consultants and the Carolina Global Breastfeeding Institute

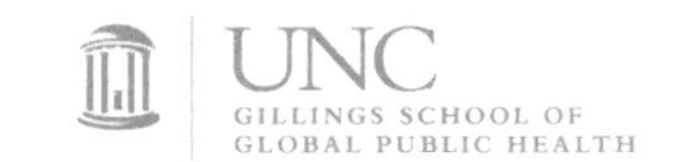

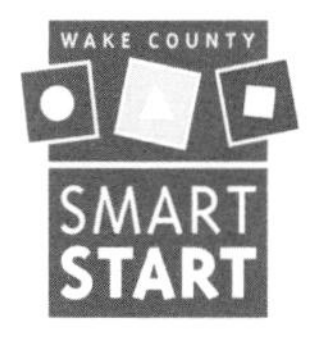

Child Care Health Consultant Program is funded by Wake County SmartStart, working to ensure children, ages 0 to 5, are prepared for success in school and in life.

Nutritionist/Registered Dietitian, Consultant, and Food Service Staff Qualifications

TITLE	LEVEL OF PROFESSIONAL RESPONSIBILITY	EDUCATION AND EXPERIENCE
Nutritionist/ Registered Dietitian/ Child Care Nutrition Consultant (state level)	Develops policies and procedures for implementation of nutrition food standards statewide and provides consultation to state agency personnel, including staff involved with licensure.	Current registration with the Commission on Dietetic Registration of the American Dietetic Association or eligibility for registration with a Bachelor's and Master's degree in nutrition (including or supplemented by course(s) in child growth and development), plus at least two years of related experience as a Nutritionist or Dietitian in a health program, including services to infants and children, is preferred. Training and experience in the specific needs of children and infants is necessary. A Master's degree from an approved program in public health nutrition may be substituted for registration with the Commission on Dietetic Registration. Current state licensure or certification as a Nutritionist or Dietitian is acceptable.
Nutritionist/Registered Dietitian (local level)	Provides expertise to the early care and education director and provides ongoing guidance, consultation, and inservice training to facility's nutrition component. The number of sites and facilities for one child care Nutritionist/Registered Dietitian will vary according to size and complexity of local facilities.	Registered Dietitian, as above. At least one year of experience as described above.
Food Service Manager	Has overall supervisory responsibility for the food service unit at one or more facility sites.	High school diploma or GED. Successful completion of a food handler/food protection class. Coursework in basic menu-planning skills, basic foods, introduction to child feeding programs for managers, and/or other relevant courses (offered at community colleges). Two years of food service experience.
Food Service Worker (Cook)	Under the supervision of the Food Service Manager, carries out food service operations including menu planning, food preparation and service, and related duties in a designated area.	High school diploma or GED. Successful completion of a food handler/food protection class. Coursework in basic menu-planning skills and basic foods (offered through adult education or a community college). One year of food service experience.
Food Service Aide	Works no more than four hours a day, under the supervision of an employee at a higher level in food service unit.	High school diploma or GED. Must pass the food handler test within one to two months of employment. No prior experience is required for semi-skilled persons who perform assigned tasks in designated areas.

GLOSSARY

See Also **Acronyms** (Page 70)

Note: Some of these definitions were contained in the first edition of *Caring for Our Children* in which they were reprinted with permission from Infectious Diseases in Child Care Settings: Information for Directors, Caregivers, and Parents or Guardians, by the Epidemiology Departments of Hennepin County Community Health, St. Paul Division of Public Health, Minnesota Department of Health, Washington County Public Health, and Bloomington Division of Health. Other definitions are from the resources referenced at the end of the definition. Others were supplied by our Technical Panels.

Aflatoxin - A naturally occurring mycotoxin (fungus) produced by mold. The mold occurs in soil, decaying vegetation, hay, and grains undergoing microbiological deterioration. Favorable conditions include high moisture content and high temperature (USDA).

Age-appropriate solid foods - Also known as complementary foods, foods introduced at age-appropriate levels to infants. Examples are iron-fortified infant cereals and pureed meats for infants.

Allergens - A substance (food, pollen, pets, mold, medication, etc.) that causes an allergic reaction.

Anaphylaxis - A fungus that is most commonly found in corn, cotton, peanuts, and tree nuts. Moisture, insects, and high temperatures can cause aflatoxin crop damage. Growth is most commonly found when a period of drought is followed by a period of high humidity. Aflatoxin can also attack crops during storage or if drying is delayed. Rodents and insects can also cause contamination. Ref: U.S. Department of Agriculture, Risk Management Agency. 2008. A Risk Management Agency fact sheet: Loss adjustment procedures for aflatoxin. Rev. ed. http://www.rma.usda.gov/pubs/2005/aflatoxinfactsheet.pdf.

Anemia - Having too little hemoglobin (hemoglobin carries oxygen from the lungs throughout the body). The terms anemia, iron deficiency, and iron deficiency anemia often are used interchangeably. Iron deficiency ranges from depleted iron stores without functional or health impairment to iron deficiency with anemia, which affects the functioning of several organ systems. Ref: Centers for Disease Control and Prevention. 2007. Iron deficiency. http://www.cdc.gov/nccdphp/dnpa/nutrition/nutrition_for_everyone/iron_deficiency/index.htm.

Aspiration - The inhalation of food, liquid, or a foreign body into a person's airway, possibly resulting in choking and respiratory distress.

Assessment - An in-depth appraisal conducted to diagnose a condition or determine the importance or value of a procedure.

Bacteria (Plural of bacterium) - Organisms that may be responsible for localized or generalized diseases and can survive in and out of the body. They are much larger than viruses and can usually be treated effectively with antibiotics.

BMI - See Body Mass Index

Body fluids - Urine, feces, saliva, blood, nasal discharge, eye discharge, and injury or tissue discharge.

Body Mass Index (BMI) - Weight in kilograms divided by height in meters squared. Overweight and obesity can be defined by the BMI for age measurement. Ref: Hagan, J. F., J. S. Shaw, P. M. Duncan. 2008. *Bright futures: Guidelines for health supervision of infants, children and adolescents*. 3rd ed. Elk Grove Village, IL: American Academy of Pediatrics.

Bottle propping - Bottle-feeding an infant by propping the bottle near the infant's mouth and leaving the infant alone rather than holding the bottle by hand.

Botulism - A neuroparalytic disorder characterized by an acute, afebrile, symmetric, descending flaccid paralysis. Paralysis is caused by blockade of neurotransmitter at the voluntary motor and autonomic neuromuscular junctions. Three distinct, naturally occurring forms of human botulism exist: foodborne, wound, and infant. Ref: Pickering, L., ed. 2009. *Red Book: 2009 report of the Committee on Infectious Diseases*. 28th ed. Elk Grove Village, IL: American Academy of Pediatrics.

BPA (BISPHENOL A) - Used to manufacture polycarbonate plastics. This type of plastic is used to make some types of beverage containers, compact disks, plastic dinnerware, impact-resistant safety equipment, automobile parts, and toys. BPA epoxy resins are used in the protective linings of food cans, in dental sealants, and in other products. Ref: Centers for Disease Control and Prevention. 2009. National report on human exposure to environmental chemicals. Fact sheet: Bisphenol A. http://www.cdc.gov/exposurereport/BisphenolA_FactSheet.html.

Care Plan - A document that provides specific health care information, including any medications, procedures, precautions, or adaptations to diet or environment that may be needed to care for a child with chronic medical conditions or special health care needs. Care plans also describe signs and symptoms of impending illness and outline the response needed to those signs and symptoms. A care plan is completed by the primary care provider and should be updated on a regular basis. Ref: Donoghue, E. A., C. A. Kraft, eds. 2010. *Managing chronic health needs in child care and schools: A quick reference guide*. Elk Grove Village, IL: American Academy of Pediatrics.

Caregiver/Teacher - The primary staff who works directly with the children, that is, teacher, aide, or others in a center and the early care and education provider in a small and large family child care home.

Celiac Disease - A digestive disease that damages the small intestine and interferes with absorption of nutrients from food. People who have celiac disease cannot tolerate gluten, a protein in wheat, rye, and barley. Gluten is found mainly in foods but may also be found in everyday products such as medicines, vitamins, and lip balms. Ref: National Digestive Diseases Information Clearinghouse. 2008. Celiac disease. http://digestive.niddk.nih.gov/ddiseases/pubs/celiac/#what.

Child and Adult Care Food Program (CACFP) - The U.S. Department of Agriculture's sponsored program whose early care and education component provides nutritious meals to children enrolled in centers and family child care homes throughout the country.

Child Care Health Consultant - A licensed health professional with education and experience in child and community health and early care and education plus specialized training in child care health consultation.

Child:staff ratio - The amount of staff required, based on the number of children present and the ages of these children.

Children with special health care needs - Children who have or are at increased risk for chronic physical, developmental, behavioral, or emotional conditions who require health and related services of a type or amount beyond that required by children generally. Ref: Maternal and Child Health Bureau. Achieving and Measuring Success: A National Agenda for Children with Special Health Care Needs http://mchb.hrsa.gov/programs/specialneeds/measuresuccess.htm.

Chronic - Describing a disease or illness of long duration or frequent recurrence, often having a slow progressive course of indefinite duration. Ref: Merriam-Webster. 2010. Chronic. Medline Plus Medical Dictionary. http://www.merriam-webster.com/medlineplus/chronic.

Clean - To remove dirt and debris by scrubbing and washing with a detergent solution and rinsing with water.

Complementary foods - Solid foods that are age appropriate for infants such as iron-fortified infant cereals and pureed meats.

Compliance - The act of carrying out a recommendation, policy, regulation or procedure.

Contamination - The presence of infectious microorganisms in or on the body, on environmental surfaces, on articles of clothing, or in food or water.

"Cue" feeding - The caregiver/teacher is alert to the infant and child's cues and feeds based on those rather than teach the infant they must "demand" (cry) for their food.

Dental caries - Tooth decay resulting in localized destruction of tooth tissue. Also known as dental cavities.

Diabetes - A group of diseases marked by high levels of blood glucose resulting from defects in insulin production, insulin action, or both. Ref: National Diabetes Education Program. The facts about diabetes: America's seventh leading cause of death. http://www.ndep.nih.gov/diabetes-facts/index.aspx.

Diarrhea - An increased number of abnormally loose stools in comparison with the individual's usual bowel habits.

Disinfect - To destroy or inactivate any germs on any inanimate object.

Dyslipidemia – A condition marked by abnormal concentrations of lipids or lipoproteins in the blood, consisting of one or a combination of high LDL, low HDL, and high triglycerides.

***E. coli* 0157:H7** - One of hundreds of strains of *Escherichia coli*. Although most strains are harmless and live in the intestines of healthy humans and animals, this strain produces a powerful toxin and can cause severe illness, including bloody diarrhea and abdominal cramps. Eating undercooked meat, drinking unpasteurized milk, and swimming in or drinking sewage-contaminated water can cause infection.

Epidemic - Affecting or tending to affect an atypically large number of individuals within a population, community, or region at the same time. Ref: Merriam-Webster. 2010. Epidemic. Medline Plus Medical Dictionary. http://www.merriam-webster.com/medlineplus/epidemic.

EpiPen - An automatic epinephrine injector. Epinephrine is administered in response to some allergic reactions. Ref: Donoghue, E.A., C.A. Kraft, editors.2009. *Managing chronic health needs in child care and schools*. Elk Grove Village, IL: American Academy of Pediatrics.

Ergot - A toxic fungus found as a parasite on grains of rye and other grains. Consumption of food contaminated with ergots may cause vomiting, diarrhea and may lead to gangrene in serious cases. Chronic exposure through consumption of contaminated food can lead to health complications.

Evaluation - Impressions and recommendations formed after a careful appraisal and study.

Facilitated play - To engage children in appropriate play experiences that facilitate development in all domains and promote autonomy, competency and a sense of joy in discovery and learning. Ref: Liske, V., L. Bell. Play and the impaired child. http://www.playworks.net/article-play-and-impaired-child.html

Facility - The buildings, the grounds, the equipment, and the people involved in providing early care and education of any type.

Foodborne illness/disease - An illness or disease transmitted through food products.

Free play - See Unstructured physical activity

Galactosemia - A condition in which the body is unable to use (metabolize) the simple sugar galactose. Ref: Medline Plus. 2009. Galactosemia. Medical Encyclopedia. http://www.nlm.nih.gov/medlineplus/ency/article/000366.htm.

Gastric tube feeding - The administration of nourishment through a tube that has been surgically inserted directly into the stomach.

Gross motor skills - Large movements involving the arms, legs, feet, or the entire body (such as crawling, running, and jumping).

Group size - The number of children assigned to a caregiver/teacher or team of caregivers/teachers occupying an individual classroom or well defined space within a larger room. See also Child:Staff Ratio.

Health advocate – In early care and education settings, caregivers/teachers who spend several hours a week with specific duties designed to promote the health and safety of children in their care. They receive special training to prevent, recognize, and correct health and safety problems in early childhood education programs. The health advocate does not fill the same role as the child care health consultant. See also definition for Child Care Health Consultant. Ref: California Childcare Health Program. 2006. *Instructor's guide: The role of the child care health advocate*. University of California, San Francisco School of Nursing, Department of Family Health Care Nursing. http://www.ucsfchildcarehealth.org/pdfs/Curricula/Instsuctors_Guide/CCHA_IG_2_Role_v3.pdf

Health care professional - A person who by education, training, certification, or licensure is qualified to and is engaged in providing health care. Ref: http://medical-dictionary.thefreedictionary.com/Health+care+professional

Health consultant - See Child Care Health Consultant

Health Plan - See Care Plan.

Hepatitis - Inflammation of the liver caused by viral infection. There are six types of infectious hepatitis: type A; type B; nonA, nonB; C; and D.

Human Immunodeficiency Virus (HIV) disease - The virus that can lead to acquired immune deficiency syndrome, or AIDS. HIV damages a person's body by destroying specific blood cells, called CD4+ T cells, which are crucial to helping the body fight diseases. Ref: Centers for Disease Control and Prevention. 2006. HIV/AIDS Basics: What is HIV? http://www.cdc.gov/hiv/resources/qa/definitions.htm.

Hypercholesterolemia - Having elevated cholesterol levels. High levels of cholesterol increase the risk for cardiovascular disease and stroke.

Infant - A child between the time of birth and the age of ambulation (usually the ages from birth through twelve months).

Infection - A condition caused by the multiplication of an infectious agent in the body. Ref: Aronson, S. S., T. R. Shope, eds. 2009. *Managing infectious diseases in child care and schools: A quick reference guide*, 2nd edition. Elk Grove Village, IL: American Academy of Pediatrics.

Ingestion - The act of taking material (whether food or other substances) into the body through the mouth.

Kinesiology – The study of the principles of mechanics and anatomy in relation to human movement. Ref: Merriam-Webster. 2010. Kinesiology. Merriam-Webster Online. http://www.merriam-webster.com/dictionary/kinesiology.

Lecithin - Any of several waxy lipids which are widely distributed in animals and plants, and have emulsifying, wetting, and antioxidant properties.

Lymphoma - A general term for a group of cancers that originate in the lymph system. The two primary types of lymphoma are Hodgkin lymphoma, which spreads in an orderly manner from one group of lymph nodes to another; and non-Hodgkin lymphoma, which spreads through the lymphatic system in a non-orderly manner. Ref: Centers for Disease Control and Prevention. 2009. Hematologic (blood) cancers: Lymphoma. http://www.cdc.gov/cancer/hematologic/lymphoma/.

Medical home - Primary care that is accessible, continuous, comprehensive, family centered, coordinated, compassionate, and culturally effective. The child health care professional/primary care provider works in partnership with the family and patient to ensure that all the medical and non-medical needs of the patient are met. Ref: Hagan, J. F., J. S. Shaw, P. M. Duncan. 2008. *Bright futures: Guidelines for health supervision of infants, children and adolescents*. 3rd ed. Elk Grove Village, IL: American Academy of Pediatrics.

Medications - Any substance that is intended to cure, treat, or prevent disease or is intended to affect the structure or function of the body of humans or other animals.

Morbidity - The incidence of a disease within a population. Ref: Aronson, S. S., T. R. Shope, eds. 2009. *Managing infectious diseases in child care and schools: A quick reference guide*, 2nd edition. Elk Grove Village, IL: American Academy of Pediatrics.

Motor skills - Coordinated muscle movements involved in movement, object control, and postural control perceived as occurring after a stage (or stages) involving birth reflexes, with the idea that fundamental motor skills must be mastered before development of more sport-specific skills. Ref: Barnett, L. M., E. van Beurden, P. J. Morgan, L. O. Brooks, J. R. Beard. 2009. Childhood motor skill proficiency as a predictor of adolescent physical activity. *J Adolescent Health* 44:252-9.

Nasogastric tube feeding - The administration of nourishment using a plastic tube that stretches from the nose to the stomach.

Necrotizing enterocolitis - A condition when the lining of the intestinal wall dies and the tissue falls off. The cause for this disorder is unknown. However, it is thought that a decrease in blood flow to the bowel keeps the bowel from producing mucus that protects the gastrointestinal tract. Bacteria in the intestine may also be a cause. This disorder usually develops in an infant that is already ill or premature, and most often develops while the infant is still in the hospital. Ref: Medline Plus. 2009. Necrotizing enterocolitis. Medical Encyclopedia. http://www.nlm.nih.gov/medlineplus/ency/article/001148.htm.

Nutritionist/Registered Dietitian - A professional with one to two years' experience in infant and child health programs and coursework in child development, who serves as local or state consultant to early care and education staff.

Obesity - Obesity is an excess percentage of body weight (Body Mass Index equal or greater than 95%) due to fat that puts people at risk for many health problems. In children older than two years of age, obesity is assessed by a measure called the Body Mass Index (BMI). Ref: American Academy of Pediatrics. About childhood obesity. http://www.aap.org/obesity/about.html.

Occupational therapy - Treatment based on the engagement in meaningful activities of daily life of a typical child (such as play, feeding, toileting, and dressing). Child specific exercises are developed in order to encourage a child with mental or physical disabilities to contribute to their own recovery and development.

Organisms - Living things. Often used as a general term for germs (such as bacteria, viruses, fungi, or parasites) that can cause disease.

OSHA - Abbreviation for the Occupational Safety and Health Administration of the U.S. Department of Labor, which regulates health and safety in the workplace.

Overweight - Children and adolescents with a BMI equal to or over the 85th percentile for age but less than the 95th percentile for age are considered overweight. Ref: American Academy of Pediatrics. About childhood obesity. http://www.aap.org/obesity/about.html.

Parasite - An organism that lives on or in another living organism (such as ticks, lice, mites).

Parent/Guardian - The child's natural or adoptive mother or father, or other legally responsible person.

Pasteurized - The partial sterilization of a food substance and especially a liquid (as milk) at a temperature and for a period of exposure that destroys objectionable organisms without major chemical alteration of the substance. Ref: Merriam-Webster. 2010. Pasteurization. Merriam-Webster Online. http://www.merriam-webster.com/dictionary/pasteurization.

Perishable Foods - Foods (such as fruit, vegetables, meat, milk and dairy, and eggs) that are liable to spoil or decay. Ref: Merriam-Webster. 2010. Perishable. Merriam-Webster Online. http://www.merriam-webster.com/dictionary/perishable.

Phenylketonuria (PKU) - A genetic disorder in which the body can't process part of a protein called phenylalanine (Phe). Phe is in almost all foods. If the Phe level gets too high, it can damage the brain and cause severe mental retardation. All infants born in U.S. hospitals must now have a screening test for PKU. Ref: National Institute of Child Health and Human Development. 2009. Phenylketonuria. Medline Plus. http://www.nlm.nih.gov/medlineplus/phenylketonuria.html.

Phthalates - A group of chemicals used to make plastics more flexible and harder to break. They are often called plasticizers. They are used in products, such as vinyl, adhesives, detergents, oils, plastics, and personal-care products. Ref: National Report on Human Exposure to Environmental Chemicals. 2009. Fact sheet: Phthalates. Centers for Disease Control and Prevention. http://www.cdc.gov/exposurereport/Phthalates_FactSheet.html.

Physical activity - Any bodily movement produced by the contraction of skeletal muscle that increases energy expenditure above a basal level. Physical activity generally refers to the subset of activity that enhances health. Ref: National Center for Chronic Disease Prevention and Health Promotion. 2008. Physical activity for everyone: Glossary of terms. Centers for Disease Control and Prevention. http://www.cdc.gov/physicalactivity/everyone/glossary/index.html.

Physical therapy - The use of physical agents and methods (such as massage, therapeutic exercises, hydrotherapy, electrotherapy) to assist a child with physical or mental disabilities to optimize their individual physical development or to restore their normal body function after illness or injury.

Pica - A pattern of eating non-food materials (such as dirt or paper). Ref: Medline Plus. 2008. Pica. Medical Encyclopedia. http://www.nlm.nih.gov/medlineplus/ency/article/001538.htm.

Polybrominated diphenyl ethers (PBDE) – Flame-retardant chemicals added to plastics and foam products to make them difficult to burn. Because they are mixed into plastics and foams rather than bound to them, PBDEs can leave the products that contain them and enter the environment. Ref: Agency for Toxic Substances and Disease Registry. 2004. ToxFAQs for Polybrominated diphenyl ethers (PBDEs). http://www.atsdr.cdc.gov/tfacts68-pbde.html.

Preschooler - A child between the age of toilet learning/training and the age of entry into a regular school; usually three to five years of age.

Primary care provider - A person who by education, training, certification, or licensure is qualified to and is engaged in providing health care. A primary care provider coordinates the care of a child with the child's specialist and therapists . Ref: Donoghue, E. A., C. A. Kraft, eds. 2010. *Managing chronic health needs in child care and schools: A quick reference guide.* Elk Grove Village, IL: American Academy of Pediatrics.

Reflux - An abnormal backward flow of stomach contents into the esophagus.

Salmonella - A type of bacteria that causes food poisoning (salmonellosis) with symptoms of vomiting, diarrhea, and abdominal pain.

Salmonellosis - A diarrheal infection caused by Salmonella bacteria.

Sanitize - A process that reduces germs on inanimate surfaces to levels considered safe by public health codes or regulations.

School-age child - This term describes a developmental period associated with a child who is enrolled in a regular school, including kindergarten; usually from five to eighteen years of age. For the purposes of early care and education settings, the maximum age is usually twelve years of age.

Screen time - Time spent watching TV, videotapes, or DVDs; playing video or computer games; and surfing the internet. Ref: Guide to Community Preventive Services. 2010. *Obesity prevention: Behavioral interventions to reduce screen time.* http://www.thecommunityguide.org/obesity/behavioral.html.

Sedentary activity - Non-moving activity like reading, playing a board game, or drawing. Sedentary activity does not provide much physical activity and/or exercise. Ref.: Nemours Health and Prevention Services. 2009. *Best practices for physical activity: A guide to help children grow up healthy – For organizations serving children and youth.* Newark, DE: Nemours Health and Prevention Services. http://static.nemours.org/www-filebox/nhps/grow-up-healthy/pa-guidelines-2009.pdf.

SIDS - See Sudden Infant Death Syndrome

Staff - Used here to indicate all personnel employed at the facility, including both caregivers/teachers and personnel who do not provide direct care to the children (such as administrators, cooks, drivers, and housekeeping personnel).

Structured physical activity - Caregiver/teacher-led, developmentally appropriate, and fun. Structured activity should include:

- Daily planned physical activity that supports age-appropriate motor skill development. The activity should be engaging and involve all children with minimal or no waiting.
- Daily, fun physical activity that is vigorous (gets children "breathless" or breathing deeper and faster than during typical activities) for short bouts of time.

Ref: Nemours Health and Prevention Services. 2009. *Best practices for physical activity: A guide to help children grow up healthy – For organizations serving children and youth*. Newark, DE: Nemours Health and Prevention Services. http://static.nemours.org/www-filebox/nhps/grow-up-healthy/pa-guidelines-2009.pdf.

Sudden Infant Death Syndrome (SIDS) - The sudden death of an infant less than one year of age that cannot be explained after a thorough investigation is conducted, including a complete autopsy, examination of the death scene, and review of the clinical history. Ref: Centers for Disease Control and Prevention. 2009. Sudden Infant Death Syndrome (SIDS) and Sudden Unexpected Infant Death (SUID): Home. http://www.cdc.gov/SIDS/index.htm.

Toddler - A child between the age of ambulation and the age of toilet learning/training, usually thirteen through thirty-five months of age.

Toxoplasmosis - A parasitic disease often causing no symptoms. When symptoms do occur, swollen glands, fatigue, malaise, muscle pain, fluctuating low fever, rash, headache, and sore throat are reported most commonly. Toxoplasmosis can infect and damage a fetus while producing mild or no symptoms in the mother.

Transmission - The passing of an infectious organism or germ from person to person.

Ulcerative colitis - A disease that causes inflammation and sores, called ulcers, in the lining of the rectum and colon. Ulcers form where inflammation has killed the cells that usually line the colon, then bleed and produce pus. Inflammation in the colon also causes the colon to empty frequently, causing diarrhea. Ref: National Institute of Diabetes and Digestive and Kidney Diseases. 2006. Ulcerative colitis. http://digestive.niddk.nih.gov/ddiseases/pubs/colitis/.

Unstructured physical activity - Child-led free play. Unstructured activity should include:

- Activities that respect and encourage children's individual abilities and interests.
- Caregiver/teacher engagement with children, support for extending play, and gentle prompts and encouragement by caregivers/teachers, when appropriate, to stay physically active.

Ref: Nemours Health and Prevention Services. 2009. *Best practices for physical activity: A guide to help children grow up healthy – For organizations serving children and youth*. Newark, DE: Nemours Health and Prevention Services. http://static.nemours.org/www-filebox/nhps/grow-up-healthy/pa-guidelines-2009.pdf.

Vegetarian - There are various degrees of vegetarianism. Although none eat meat, poultry, or fish, there are other areas in which they vary. Lacto-ovo-vegetarians consume eggs, dairy products, and plant foods and lacto-vegetarians eat dairy products and plant foods but not eggs. Ref: Healthy Children. 2010. Vegetarian diets for children. American Academy of Pediatrics. http://www.healthychildren.org/English/ages-stages/gradeschool/nutrition/pages/Vegetartian-Diet-for-Children.aspx?nfstatus=401&nftoken=00000000-0000-0000-0000-000000000000&nfstatusdescription=ERROR:+No+local+token.

Vegan - Individual does not eat meat, poultry, fish, eggs, or dairy products, only plant foods. Ref: Healthy Children. 2010. Vegetarian diets for children. American Academy of Pediatrics. http://www.healthychildren.org/English/ages-stages/gradeschool/nutrition/pages/Vegetartian-Diet-for-Children.aspx?nfstatus=401&nftoken=00000000-0000-0000-0000-000000000000&nfstatusdescription=ERROR:+No+local+token.

Viandas - Root vegetables common in some Hispanic diets. Ref: Block, G., P. Wakimoto, C. Jensen, S. Mandel, R. R. Green. 2006. Validation of a food frequency questionnaire for Hispanics. *Preventing Chronic Disease* 3(3): 1-10. http://www.cdc.gov/pcd/issues/2006/jul/pdf/05_0219.pdf.

Vigorous-intensity physical activity - Rhythmic, repetitive physical activity that uses large muscle groups, causing a child to breathe rapidly and only enabling them to speak in short phrases. Typically children's heart rates are substantially increased and they are likely to be sweating. Ref. Nemours Health and Prevention Services. 2009. *Best practices for physical activity: A guide to help children grow up healthy – For organizations serving children and youth*. Newark, DE: Nemours Health and Prevention Services. http://static.nemours.org/www-filebox/nhps/grow-up-healthy/pa-guidelines-2009.pdf.

Virus - A microscopic organism, smaller than a bacterium, that may cause disease. Viruses can grow or reproduce only in living cells.

WIC - Abbreviation for the U.S. Department of Agriculture's Special Supplemental Food Program for Women, Infants and Children, which provides food supplements and nutrition education to pregnant and breastfeeding women, infants, and young children who are considered to be at nutritional risk due to their level of income and evidence of inadequate diet.

ACRONYMS/ABBREVIATIONS USED

AAFP – American Academy of Family Physicians

AAP – American Academy of Pediatrics

AAPD – American Academy of Pediatric Dentistry

ABM – Academy of Breastfeeding Medicine

ACS – American Cancer Society

ADA – American Diabetes Association

ADA – American Dietetic Association

AHA – American Heart Association

AIDS – Acquired Immunodeficiency Syndrome

APHA – American Public Health Association

BMI – Body Mass Index

BPA – Bisphenol A

CACFP – Child and Adult Care Food Program

CCHC – Child Care Health Consultant

CDC – Centers for Disease Control and Prevention

CFOC – *Caring for Our Children: National Health and Safety Performance Standards; Guidelines for Early Care and Education Programs*

CFR – Code of Federal Regulations

CSHCN – Children with Special Health Care Needs

EMS – Emergency Medical Services

EPA – U.S. Environmental Protection Agency

FDA – U.S. Food and Drug Administration

HBV – Hepatitis B Virus

HCV – Hepatitis C Virus

HIV – Human Immunodeficiency Virus

HMRS – Healthy Meals Resource System

HRSA – U.S. Health Resources and Services Administration

IU – International units

MCHB – Maternal and Child Health Bureau

NAP-SACC – Nutrition and Physical Activity Self-assessment for Child Care

NASPE – National Association for Sport and Physical Education

NEC – Necrotizing enterocolitis

NFSMI – National Food Service Management Institute

NRC – National Resource Center for Health and Safety in Child Care and Early Education

NWS – National Weather Service

OSHA – Occupational Safety and Health Administration

PBDE – Polybrominated diphenyl ethers

PC – Polycarbonate

SIDS – Sudden infant death syndrome

SNE – Society for Nutrition Education

UNICEF – United Nations Children's Fund

USBC – United States Breastfeeding Committee

USDA – U.S. Department of Agriculture

WIC – Women, Infants, and Children

WHO – World Health Organization

INDEX

G

H

I

J

L

M

N

O

P

Q

R

S

T

U

V

W

Y

***Bold** number within a listing represents primary discussion of topic*